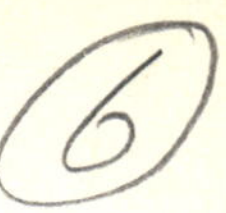

AF566674

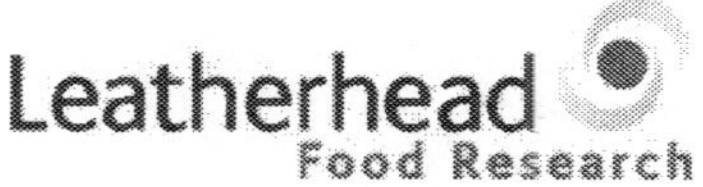

FOOD CHAIN ALLERGEN MANAGEMENT

Proceedings of a conference held at
Leatherhead Food Research
20 May 2009

Edited by

Victoria Emerton

RSC Publishing

This edition first published 2009 by
Leatherhead Publishing, a division of
Leatherhead Food International Ltd
Randalls Road, Leatherhead, Surrey KT22 7RY, UK
URL: http://www.leatherheadfood.com

and

Royal Society of Chemistry
Thomas Graham House, Science Park, Milton Road,
Cambridge, CB4 0WF, UK
URL: http://www.rsc.org
Regstered Charity No. 207890

Special Publication No 329

Proceedings of a conference held at
Leatherhead Food Research
20 May 2009

ISBN: 978-1-905224-85-2

A catalogue record of this book is available from the British Library

Printed in Great Britain by the MPG Books Group, Bodmin and King's Lynn

CONTENTS

CONTRIBUTORS

Biographies

David Highton

David Highton is the British Standards Institution's Group Scheme Manager with responsibility for Food and Social Accountability Schemes. His role is to provide the Group technical focus for the management of accreditation, technical compliance and certification. Before joining BSI in 1998 David spent over 25 years in Trading Standards. His interest in allergens and food safety management controls of allergens comes from this breadth of experience in associated regulatory enforcement and management and production control assessment and certification. Through this experience and several recommendations David was invited to sit on the Allergy Standard Technical Committee.

Sue Hattersley

Sue Hattersley has been Head of the Food Allergy Branch at the Food Standards Agency since 2002. She is responsible for all aspects of food allergy and food intolerance (other than diagnosis and clinical management), including statutory and voluntary labelling, as well as raising awareness of food allergy and intolerance issues with food businesses, enforcement bodies and other stakeholders. She is also responsible for a significant research programme that underpins the development of Agency policy in this area. Sue's background is in toxicology, originally working in the pharmaceutical industry before moving into Department of Health, where she worked on the safety of food chemicals and then novel foods. She moved from DH into the Agency when it was formed in 2000.

Tony Hines

Tony Hines has run Crisis Management Consultancy services and training courses in the UK, Spain, Ireland and around the world. Private clients include many of Europe's top ten food and drinks manufacturers. Over the last three years Tony has worked closely with the Food Standards Agency, Industry and Retailers on incident management and communication within a number of specific product categories. He has over 20 years experience in delivering training programs in a lively and unforgettable format and has worked at Leatherhead for over 35 years. He has delivered conference presentations on Crisis and Incident Management around the world. Tony has written a number of journal articles and has contributed to several authoritative works on Crisis Management.

Neil Griffiths

Neil Griffiths has worked for over thirty years advising the Consumer Product Industry on brand protection. This he achieved by supplying the necessary support to enable the industry to meet the constantly changing legislative requirements to produce safe, compositionally correct, environmentally friendly, properly labelled products. This was initially undertaken through his roles within the UK enforcement authorities, but since 1987 through his company Lawlabs of which he was the principal founder. In 2005 he sold Lawlabs to Bodycote plc and since that time he has continued to provide consultancy support to the food industry through his consultancy practice Neil Griffiths Consultants. Neil has provided consultancy support to the Anaphylaxis Campaign (AC) over the past 5 years and was co author of the AC Manufacturing and Catering Standards and Guidance.

Geoff Spriegel

Geoff has extensive experience in Food Safety and Quality management based on over 30 years experience with major companies such as St Ivel, Diageo and Sainsbury's. In the last 5 years he has worked as a consultant to Food and Drink manufacturers and Retailers and has also undertaken project work for the Food Standards Agency. Geoff is currently engaged by the British Retail Consortium to develop the international potential of the BRC Global Standards Schemes for Food, Packaging, Storage and Distribution and Consumer Products.

Deryck Tremble

Deryck has worked for 14 years for AIB International, he began as an auditor and has now been Regional General Manager - Europe, Africa and Middle East for the last few years. Previously he worked for Allied Domecq, Kraft, Unilever and ABF in Production and Quality Management Roles. He has audited facilities and trained personnel all over the world. He speaks at many seminars and enjoys highlighting the importance of Food Safety and Allergen Management.

John Figgins

For the past 9 nine years John has been Chemistry Manager at Sainsbury's Supermarkets Ltd – a role that covers all aspects of chemical food safety including allergen control policy & practice. Prior to joining Sainsbury's he was employed as an analyst at the Laboratory of the Government Chemist working in a number of departments including food analysis, analysis of animal products for veterinary residues and research into the chemical hazards of tobacco smoke. His degree was in Applied Chemistry.

Terry Wilde

Terry is the Product Integrity Manager at Tesco Stores Ltd. He works within the Supply Chain Technology Team in Tesco's Trading Law and Technical

Department. Terry has a degree in Food Technology from the University of Reading. Since graduating, Terry has 18 years experience in food manufacturing across a range of product sectors. Terry joined Tesco just over one year ago and has been responsible for the implementation of the Tesco Food Manufacturing Standard across the entire Tesco supply base. Terry has recently overseen the launch and implementation of the Tesco Non-Food Standard. In his role within the Supply Chain Technology Team, Terry has the responsibility of setting Tesco Group manufacturing standards which includes allergen management.

Moira Howie

Moira studied Nutrition with Biology and has worked in the retail industry for the past 13 years. She joined Waitrose 5 years ago to develop and deliver an integrated health & nutrition policy and a customer facing Nutrition Advice Service. Moira sits on the Editorial board of the British Nutrition Foundation and has chaired two working groups for the Institute of Grocery Distribution one on Packaging Legibility and more recently Saturated Fat Communication: Enabling Consumers to Make More Informed Choices.

Jacqueline Ross

Jac Ross has worked for Marks and Spencer as a Food Technologist for 9 years. As part of her role within Marks and Spencer she chairs the Allergen Working Group - one of 3 Food Safety Groups advising the Food Division on policy relating to allergen management within Marks and Spencer Stores and their supply base. Prior to Marks and Spencer, Jac worked in various technical and innovation roles for Natures Way Foods, Uniq Prepared Foods and Unilever Food Solutions

Simon Flanagan

Simon is Head of RSSL's Specialty Analysis Division and heads up technical services in the field of allergens. He has worked in various sectors of the food industry for over twenty years. Simon has worked with two of the largest UK contract analytical laboratories, where he has been instrumental in establishing and validating dedicated allergen testing laboratories and consultancy based services for the food industry.

Clare Mills

Clare Mills studied Biochemistry at the University of Bristol, UK and then went on to study for a PhD Biochemistry at the University of Kent at Canterbury. For the last 10 years she has led the Food Structure and Health Group within which her personal research team has been focused on studying the role physicochemical behaviour of food structures plays the development of IgE-mediated food allergy. Clare currently leads a project worth €14.3M with 63 partners from across Europe to tackle the problems of food allergy (www.europrevall.org).

Jeremy Hall

Jeremy has worked in Bernard Matthews for nearly ten years and is currently group Technical Director. He has been Chairman of the British Poultry Council technical committee for the past twenty years, Chair of the Technical and Advisory committee of Quality British Turkey, and sits on the Assured Food Standards advisory committee. With a wide experience in added value poultry products, fresh and frozen formats, as well as sandwiches, pizza production, and baked pastry and patisserie products, the need for effective allergen strategies and controls is close to his heart.

CONTRIBUTORS

David Highton
Group Scheme Manager
BSI Management Systems - UK
PO Box 9000
Milton Keynes
United Kingdom

Sue Hattersley
Head of Food Allergy Branch
Food Standards Agency
Aviation House
125 Kingsway
London
United Kingdom

Tony Hines MBE
Head of Knowledge Transfer and
Crisis Management Manager
Leatherhead Food Research
Randalls Road
Leatherhead
Surrey
United Kingdom

Neil Griffiths
Neil Griffiths Consultants
16 Elder Close
Brighton
United Kingdom

Dr Geoff Spriegel
Director of Global Standards and
Technical Services
British Retail Consortium
21 Dartmouth Street
Westminster
London
United Kingdom

Deryck Tremble
AIB International
PO Box 11
Leatherhead
Surrey
United Kingdom

John Figgins
Chemistry Manager
Sainsbury's Supermarkets Ltd
33 Holborn
London
United Knigdom

Terry Wilde
Technical Manager
Tesco Foods
Delamare Road
Cheshunt
Hertfordshire
United Kingdom

Moira Howie
Company Nutritionist
Waitrose Ltd
Doncastle Road
Southern Industrial Area
Bracknell
Berkshire
United Kingdom

Jacqueline Ross
Chair, Allergen Working Group
Marks & Spencer plc
Waterside House
35 North Wharf Road
London
United Kingdom

Simon Flannagan
Reading Scientific Services Ltd
Reading Science Centre
Whiteknights Campus
Pepper Lane
Reading
United Kingdom

Dr Clare Mills
Programme Leader
Food Structure and Health
Institute of Food Research,
Norwich Research Park,
Colney, Norwich,
United Kingdom

Jeremy Hall
Group Technical Director
Bernard Matthews Farms
Great Witchingham Hall
North Witchingham
Norwich
Norfolk
United Kingdom

FOREWORD

The prevalence of food allergy is known to be significant, and a particular problem in young children. While scientific research across Europe is providing valuable information on the prevalence and patterns of food allergy; the foods involved and the sorts of allergen thresholds that will trigger a response, the EU has responded with tighter regulations on food allergen labelling to help the consumer identify the allergenic ingredients in their food. The food industry must adhere to the allergen labelling regulations, but this is only of value when underpinned by a robust and comprehensive management programme for allergens in the factory.

Leatherhead Food Research in partnership with Campden BRI held the conference *Food Chain Allergen Management* in May 2009 to inform the food industry of the management tools and Standards that are available to enable an effective allergen management plan. This book contains the lectures that were given at this event, which gathered together several of the major food retailers in the UK, specialists in auditing for allergens, an expert in crisis management and product recalls, groups involved in writing standards on which the food industry can base allergen management programmes, as well as the Food Standards Agency, a major food manufacturer, and technical researchers investigating prevalence of allergy, and the effects of cleaning regimes on removal of allergens.

Sue Hattersley of the Food Standards Agency presented information on their activity and research into allergens, Dr Geoff Spriegel of the British Retail Consortium and Neil Griffiths from the Anaphylaxis Campaign provided details of their management Standards, Tony Hines from Leatherhead Food Research outlined the sequence of events that lead to allergen-related product recalls and means of managing a situation like that, Deryck Tremble from AIB International outlined the allergen auditing process, four of the major food retailers in the UK: John Figgins from Sainsbury's, Jacqueline Ross from Marks and Spencer, Moira Howie from Waitrose and Terry Wilde from Tesco presented difference aspects of their allergen management procedures, and what allergen management is expected of their suppliers. Simon Flannagan from RSSL provided results of recent research on cleaning regimes for allergens, Dr Claire Mills from the Institute of Food Research gave details of the scope and initial findings of the EuroPrevall project, and Jeremy Hall from Bernard Matthews talked about allergen hazards in the factory.

The event was run in collaboration with the Anaphylaxis Campaign and Campden BRI and the proceedings provides the reader with a useful guide to the allergen management tools currently available, and the developments in allergen thresholds that will help with allergen control monitoring and benchmarking in the future.

My thanks go to the speakers at the conference who not only delivered excellent presentations, but gave additional time to make the production of these proceedings possible.

This book is an invaluable reference material to all those involved in ingredients and process management and HACCP implementation in the food industry.

Victoria Emerton
Leatherhead Food Research
October 2009

Food allergy continues to be a very important issue for many thousands of people across the country . Reactions can sometimes be life-threatening and concern about allergens in food can significantly impact upon the quality of life for many families. It is no wonder that many sections of the UK food industry are now taking this important subject seriously. Great strides have been made to make food safe for the allergic population and to provide them with comprehensive, accurate information.

"Food Chain Allergen Management", the major conference organised during May by Leatherhead Food Research in conjunction with Campden BRI and supported by the Anaphylaxis Campaign, demonstrated the strong commitment that many within the industry have shown to addressing the problems relating to food allergy. These problems cannot be solved overnight, but the Anaphylaxis Campaign is gratified to see that life is gradually becoming easier and safer for those affected. We consider the work that we do with the food industry to be of vital importance. We strongly encourage food companies to join the Anaphylaxis Campaign as corporate members and intend to continue the extremely productive dialogue that began with the inception of the Campaign in 1994. Meanwhile you will see in this volume examples of the high-quality thinking that already exists and which, if examined carefully, may lead to some of the solutions that industry is looking for.

Lynne Regent, Chief Executive,
Anaphylaxis Campaign

INTRODUCTION

David Highton
Global Scheme Manager – Food
British Standards Institution

It is my pleasure to write the introduction to this anthology of presentations that represent the contributions made to the Food Chain Allergen Management Conference held at Leatherhead Food Research in May 2009.

As chair of the Conference that took place, I can say without hesitation that what you will read in the following chapters truly takes you on a journey through the allergen issues that impact on today's food chain from source to the consumer, who is rightly the "focus of concern".

As Tony Hines of Leatherhead Food Research says in his contribution "The Anaphylaxis Campaign AGM in 2009 demonstrated the difficulties of living with food allergy very clearly, with contributions from consumers who are facing allergy issues. Their journey, for example a family holiday starting on an aeroplane, is often a journey 'from hell to sheer hell' as they try to cope with allergen issues and cross-contamination".

An introduction is usually and hopefully the first chapter of a good read and this is a good read. With allergen management we have to consider the system or cycle of food safety management, where every action or reaction affects another aspect of the chain. With this in mind I have selected the following phrase written by Clare Mills of the Institute of Food Research in her introduction to the penultimate chapter, which, although appearing in one of the latter chapters sums up what may be in the back of your mind as you go on the journey of discovery about allergen management in the food chain.

"30 years ago, no one had ever heard of food allergies, and there certainly were not the headlines that appear in the newspapers about people dying from allergic reactions, and all the of information that has appeared on food packaging about allergens. There certainly was not a need for children to be given adrenalin pens, nor were peanuts banned from entire schools because of children with peanut allergies. The question is, what has changed?"

What has changed? Awareness has been heightened across the whole spectrum of society, from babies to the elderly, across the whole food supply chain, from primary food producers, through food processers and manufacturers, to small retailers and multinational supermarkets, government and regulatory control agencies, and ultimately to the knowledge of the impact of specific allergens on the health of the food consumer.

The following chapters reveal in a very readable and practical approach, the key issues that are being addressed and still have to be addressed.

Knowing what the impact of allergens is on human health depends on knowing what the acceptable thresholds are, but this is still an emerging area of knowledge and study, which is explained and illustrated very succinctly. Mean while the food industry and food manufacturers soldier on in the sure and certain knowledge that they must manage and control the known food allergens and legislatively controlled ones, fully aware of managing the risks from cross contamination with food allergens, and at the same time wanting to provide meaningful and helpful information to allergic consumers. But is the information meaningful and helpful? 'May contain' advisory labels and concern over issues related to "free from". These matters are considered and addressed.

I know from my background in trading standards, food standards, and food safety management systems that even with established analytical methods for the same purpose there can be discrepancies between the analytical results; when food incidents relate to food allergens these problems are significantly prevalent, due to the issues surrounding testing for allergens. It may be that "different kits are measuring different allergens, or that different kits work better in some food matrices than others".

Broadening this theme is the chapter covering the results of a study that was run in collaboration with the Reading Scientific Services Laboratory (RSSL) and the Anaphylaxis Campaign, which monitored the effects of different cleaning methods and their ability to remove residual allergenic proteins.

Practical allergen management and control is explored further in the chapter by Jeremy Hall, Group Technical Director of Bernard Matthews Farms – "Allergens - the most vulnerable areas of a food factory". He gives manufacturers a view on how the most vulnerable "allergen" areas of food facilities should be managed. Vulnerabilities include people, engineers, product development and most of the manufacturing managers and supervisors.

For food manufacturers who need effective control of food allergens with correct labelling declarations and an understanding of their liability under EU Law, recognising these issues is significant and is addressed within several of the chapters.

With the insatiable appetite of the modern media for creating publicity on food related issues, allergy related headlines abound, and have to be considered as a significant factor in food chain allergy management not only in their own right but as a contribution related to product recall which is often not related to a direct allergen issue but to a failure in labelling control management.

Label management is of course one of many practical aspects of food safety management systems. In recent years many food safety management standards have been developed as private standards, for example the British Retail Consortium's Global Standard for Food Safety, supermarket retailers own supplier focused standards or as public standards, for example ISO22000 – Food Safety Management Systems – Requirements for any Organisation in the Food Chain and the British Standards Institution's publically available specification PAS220 – Pre-requisite Programs on Food Safety for Food Manufacturing. All of these standards to a greater or lesser extent embrace allergen control and allergen management in food production but their weakness lies in the generality with which they embrace the subject, which is why the Anaphylaxis Campaign first raised the subject of an Allergen Management Standard for the food industry in 2003. The initiative to create the Standard was started around the time of tremendously rapid changes in allergen labelling law, and challenged the food industry to adopt its principles. The standard appeared in 2007 and has set the foundations for other standards to react to and with. The digest of the chapters dealing with BRC standards, the Allergen Standard and the supermarket retailer's chapters set in context the practical issues relating to control of allergens in the manufacturing environment and dealing with controls in the retail supply chain.

Whatever food safety management system approaches are adopted, the integrity of audits and what the auditors look at and consider is a significant issue and Deryck Tremble's chapter "Allergens: Building the Foundations for a Robust Programme" covers best practices, pre-requisite programmes, and considers the control of allergens, from the practical point of view gained from surveillance activities in the food industry.

That chapter also introduces a global perspective, which for the retailers with global supply chains to administer and control impacts considerably on their perspective of allergen management and never more so than at the very interface with the "consumers" to whom they have to convey "suitable" "understandable" "legal" and "effective" allergy information.

As Moira Howie, says in her chapter "I Want It All & I Want It Now! Allergy Information for customers" - "Consumers' expectations have risen enormously; not only do they expect that all food should be safe to eat, but of course that food is safe to eat with respect to allergy information, and that information about allergens in foods is clear and concise".

This is the challenge that not only "own brand" retailers face but owners of "proprietary brands" who face similar information challenges. The several chapters by the representatives of the UK's retail supermarket chains explain how they are meeting these suppliers, labelling and information challenges from their perspectives.

A theme that develops through your read will be the importance of knowing how allergens are managed in other countries, particularly if importing or exporting is involved. Not only the technical issues and differences, but language differences which can lead to confusion: even though Americans speak English, there are distinct differences in terminology used between the two countries, and a certain amount of "translation" is required for messages to be clearly understood.

But differences don't just relate to technical and language issues. I was recently engaged in conversation with a research pharmacist who enlightened me to the fact that coatings on slow release tablets have to be varied for country to country depending on the digestive characteristics of the people involved, which in its own way brings us back to the "focus of concern"; the consumer, and the penultimate chapter which discusses the EuroPrevall project aimed at establishing how many people suffer from a food allergy in Europe, what the major foods causing food allergy are, what are the relationships between severity and minimum eliciting doses, how much of a food causes a problem, how much does it cost to society, what are the risk factors, and what is the impact on quality of life.

Food Chain Allergen Management is truly a holistic subject. No one sector of the food manufacturing or food catering industry, or private or public surveillance organisation, or food retail group dominates; everyone has an interest, everyone has a part to play, in ensuring that the impact of allergens on the health of the food consumer is increasingly understood and managed and controlled.

I am sure that as you read the following chapters you will appreciate the breadth of contributions and I hope that it will inspire you to read more, study more and understand more the whole subject of allergens and particularly management of allergens in the food chain.

1. DEVELOPMENT OF ALLERGEN MANAGEMENT THRESHOLDS

Sue Hattersley
Head of Food Allergy Branch,
Food Standards Agency

1.1 Introduction

This paper will cover a number of areas including what the Food Standards Agency has been doing in the area of allergen management, the consequences of poor allergen management, trying to draw some lessons from the incidents that have happened in the last 12 months, and what the Agency is planning to do in terms of taking forward the problem of how we determine the management threshold levels. Definition of allergen management thresholds is what the food industry is waiting for in order to be able to inform their advisory labelling decisions. Analytical methods will also be mentioned briefly.

So, as we all probably know, there is EU legislation that requires the labelling of a number of specified allergenic foods when they are used as deliberate ingredients in pre-packed foods. And this requirement, apart from sulphites, is for labelling of the deliberate ingredients, whatever the level of use, so that even the very minor ingredient at a very low level has to be labelled if it is deliberately added. However, the legislation doesn't cover the issue of allergen cross contamination, and so the situation could arise where there are higher levels of an allergen present as a result of cross contamination, which is not covered by the law and therefore may not be represented on the label of the food, whereas lower levels of an allergen which have been added deliberately as part of the product formulation do have to be labelled. In some countries the issue of cross contamination has been addressed, and if there is significant cross contamination with an allergen or allergens, then the allergens concerned can be included on the label as the last ingredient listing, but that is not permitted under EU Law. Ingredient labelling only includes an ingredient added deliberately as part of the product formulation, rather than if it is present as a cross contaminant.

1.2 Food Standards Agency Guidance Documents

The Food Standards Agency produced Best Practice Guidance on Allergen Management and Advisory Labelling in 2006 (1). This was produced once the legislation was in place covering the labelling of allergens as deliberate ingredients. The guidance was produced very much as a collaborative effort; the Food Standards Agency worked with a number of different stakeholders; the manufacturers, the retailers, the allergy support organisations, and also the enforcement bodies. This approach contributed to the success of the document because it covers a wide perspective, and is practical and helpful. The main Guidance document gives a decision tree approach to take people through allergen management. This publication is intended to help Trading Standards enforcement officers and the larger food businesses. A leaflet entitled 'Allergy – what to consider when labelling food' (2) was also produced for the smaller food businesses, which covered in outline form both the labelling requirements and the issue of allergen cross contamination. The guidance was disseminated through the stakeholders that were involved in drafting the document; so it went through the trade bodies to the industry, and through LACORS to the enforcement officers. In addition, the Agency has always provided training for enforcement officers, and so the guidance was promoted by that route to the enforcers because that was felt to be a good way to reach the smaller businesses.

This Guidance has been updated recently, because at the time it was produced, Lupin and Molluscs were not on the list of allergens that had to be labelled, and the update reflects these additions to the list of allergens for mandatory labelling.

The food industry asked the Food Standards Agency to help in the provision of clear guidance to be used across all food sectors, and this resulted in the production of these Guidance documents. The food industry was very aware of the risks from cross contamination with food allergens, and wanted to provide meaningful and helpful information to allergic consumers. At that time in 2005 there was no legislation or authoritative guidance on how to manage allergen cross contamination; the industry had different guidance documents, but there was nothing available in a cohesive form. Some guidance addressed one allergen, some addressed a few allergens. There was no consolidated picture. The food industry had no consistent approach to managing allergens, and no guidance when making decisions on when to put allergen advisory labelling on pack. Another issue relates to appropriate analytical methods for detecting and measuring the presence of allergens; if the presence of allergens in foods is going to be controlled, there need to be the analytical methods available to measure them. Analytical methods will be discussed at the end of this paper.

1.3 Warning Labelling

The Food Standards Agency was receiving a lot of information from consumers who were very confused by the advisory labelling that they were seeing on products. The different words and phrases that appear on different products were found to be confusing. Consumers also over-interpret the messages given; if labelling information is used that says there is a risk of cross contamination because nuts are also handled in the factory, the consumers will try to determine a level of risk that they think that phrase conveys. If consumers see a statement on pack that says 'made on the same production equipment', they also think that's a risk, and they will try and assign a level of risk to that. It's very clear that the labelling describes how the risk arises. However, the wording used doesn't really say anything to quantify the level of risk, but consumers judge the risk based on their own interpretation of the wording, and so they're making decisions based on the different phrases that are being used. There's also consumer concern that the labels covering the possible presence of allergens in foods are over-used, and obviously they restrict choice if consumers avoid all foods carrying warning labels. What we tend to see, particularly in teenagers, which is a group that the FSA have studied, is that they think the warning is used in order to protect the food business, and is not there to protect the consumer, and the warning is ignored because the impression is that the warnings don't mean anything. And so this leads to risk taking behaviours amongst this particular population group.

The FSA Guidance document encourages manufacturers and retailers to think about the risks of allergen cross contamination, where they might occur at any point along the food chain, whether they can be reduced or eliminated, and whether they can be managed down to a level where the risk is remote. This is encouraging the food industry to assess their production facilities and product specifications for risk, to see if they can manage that risk, and then only if that cross contamination can not be controlled down to a minimal level, to communicate that risk to the consumers. The correct procedure should be to go through the risk assessment and the allergen management stages first, and only then if there is still a risk of cross contamination with an allergen, that risk should be communicated to the consumers by means of warning labelling.

1.4 Allergen Management Thresholds

While the Guidance gives advice on best practice in allergen management and the appropriate use of warning labelling, what it doesn't do is quantify the amounts of allergens on which to base risk assessments. At the time that the Guidance was produced in 2006, it was hoped that figures could be given for the amounts of allergens required to trigger an allergic reaction, or at least an indication of management threshold levels for allergens could be included, but when the information available on allergen thresholds in the literature was studied in more detail, the science really wasn't available at that time to be able to set management levels in food to inform labelling decisions. This was partly because a lot of the information that had been published on clinical thresholds in individual patients was being produced by studies with different study designs, and with different criteria, and so it was very difficult to pull all the literature together and come to a definitive level for thresholds for the various allergens. There are now a lot of allergen challenge studies being conducted using very standard protocols and standard materials, and so we are a step or two closer to consensus on what clinical thresholds are. The next step is to translate this information from the clinical thresholds in people, through to management levels in food.

The lack of detection methods for some of the allergens is also an important issue in the allergen management area, and a key point is, that although there are detection kits available for a lot of the allergens, there are no standard reference materials. Many of the detection kits and the methods that they use are not independently validated, and this is a vital issue that needs to be addressed.

The Food Standards Agency does intend to revise its Guidance to provide quantitative information on allergen thresholds. While it would be preferable to be working on this in the next few years, it is becoming apparent that this may take longer than that for all the major food allergens.

1.5 Allergen-related Food Incidents

Allergen-related food incidents occur when allergen management goes wrong. The next section will cover what some of the common causes of allergen-related food incidents are, and the sorts of actions that businesses can take.

Looking back historically, the main cause of food allergy incidents, certainly in 2007, and perhaps at the beginning of 2008, was the wrong product being put in the wrong packet. So in situations where 2, 3, or 4 different varieties of something are being made, the packaging may not have been changed over for a new product run from the previous one, and at least at the beginning of the product run the wrong product is then in the packet, so the allergy information is completely wrong and the product needs to be withdrawn. Looking through the data for 2008 and 2009, although we did still see a significant number of cases where the product was in the wrong packet, I think this scenario is becoming less common, so businesses are getting their procedures right and getting the checks in place. There are still some incidents where there is inconsistent labelling; an allergen might be listed in the ingredients list, and while some allergens are declared in an allergy statement or box, in some cases not all of the allergens present are included in the box. This is a risk for the allergic consumer, because despite consumer education to always read the ingredients list, a lot of people use the allergy statement on products as a shortcut, and so if an allergen is missed off that statement then there's a risk because the consumer will think that product is safe for them. There have been some cases in which multipacks have allergy labelling on the outer packaging that is not consistent with the labelling on the individual products inside, and so again the consumer may just read what's on the outside, which may be right or wrong.

Looking back, most of the incidents concern deliberate ingredients and incorrect labelling, but what we are beginning to see, certainly over the last year, is more incidents related to detection of significant levels of cross contamination and this probably reflects the impact of the mandatory allergen labelling legislation that has been in place since the end of 2005. Local authorities are now doing much more sampling to check product labelling, and so they are detecting allergens in products in which the allergen is not included on the label; it's not a deliberate ingredient, but there are significant levels of cross contamination. A recent trend is with products that are described as 'free from' particular allergens where the allergen that the 'free from' statement relates to, can still be detected in the food. This is a particularly important issue, because obviously the allergic consumer has a high level of trust in 'free from' products to be suitable for them based on their particular allergy.

The FSA issued over 60 food allergy alerts in 2008, and to the middle of May 2009, there have already been 25 alerts, which is a similar level to 2008. The most common allergens involved were milk, soya, sulphites, wheat and gluten, and nuts. There were quite a lot of incidents in the last year where there were significant levels of milk cross contamination in plain chocolate products; at least half of the milk-related incidents involved milk in plain chocolate. Another trend emerging recently is in products containing dried fruit ingredients, particularly apricots, where the sulphite information is not being carried through from the ingredient through to the meal, the jam or the products that contain the apricots.

It can't be stressed enough that one of the key things to get right is to make sure that the right packaging is used for the right product. There have been incidences where the packaging either remains in the line at the end of the run and is transferred to the beginning of the next run, or perhaps the remaining packaging is put back in the packaging store, but it's not put back in the right place, so this is a very common cause of incidents. It may not be the whole batch of product that is affected by the wrong packaging, it may only be a very small number of units at the beginning of the batch that are in the wrong packet, but generally it is impossible to be sure how many individual products are affected, so the whole batch has to be withdrawn. In the case of the apricots and the sulphites, it is obviously key to get accurate information from suppliers about what allergens are in the ingredients that are being brought in to the factory, and to make sure that that information is carried through to the final product. Obviously, there should be careful consideration of where cross contamination can happen, and systems put in place to reduce this risk. Businesses that are not sure about whether their allergen management practices are sufficient, should ask for advice from their local authority. The FSA have done a lot of training for the local authority enforcement officers to help them understand allergen management practices. Enforcement officers can look at individual businesses and best advise them as to how they can manage allergens in their factory. Staff training is also a key issue; it may be that the person running the line knows what they're doing, but if that person is off sick and somebody else comes in, they may not know that line or that practice, it is key that all staff are properly trained.

The FSA has trained enforcement officers in allergen management for a number of years, and last year launched an on-line training module on allergen management, which is freely available to anybody on the Agency's website (3). Whilst this training was originally aimed at enforcement officers, it is something that, because it's freely available, is a resource that is very valuable for small businesses as it can be used from the business in a short space of time. The training is interactive, and covers the factory setting, and aspects such as packaging or cleaning.

1.6 The Future

A significant issue that the Agency is working on to take this area forward, is to consider how we might be able to set the allergen management thresholds, or action levels for allergens, that are going to lead to more consistency in the advisory labelling decisions. The other area to be addressed is validating the analytical methods that would be needed to be able to make the threshold information work.

The issues currently are: a proliferation of 'may contain' advisory labels; uncertainty from the food industry and consumers; and a lack of legislation to address allergen cross contamination. A 'risk based' approach to controlling allergens and making decisions on the advisory labelling is needed.

From the business and the consumer perspective, the key question here is how to determine the management threshold levels for use by the industry to underpin the labelling decisions - how do we move from threshold data in individual people (taking into account the question of how representative those data might be) to levels in food that are going to be protective for the allergic population. The limit of detection could be applied, and in many cases that might provide sufficient protection, but the limit of detection is going to fall as test kit methodology improves, and is not actually related to the level of risk, so whilst it could be used, it isn't a real scientifically based measurement to use in terms of risk to the consumer. If there aren't quantitative management thresholds, there will inevitably be warning labelling on foods where they are perhaps not necessary, which will lead to restriction in choice for the consumer.

From the point of view of a regulator, it would be very helpful to have some threshold levels. The legislation might need to be reviewed, because if there are very low levels of an ingredient present that has been added deliberately, that ingredient may actually not pose a risk to the allergic consumer at that level, but it is currently being declared, and so is restricting choice unnecessarily for consumers. The key thing at the moment is dealing with the food incidents involving detected levels of cross contamination. Judgements have to be made on when that level of contamination is sufficiently high that it is a risk to the allergic population, and without agreed quantitative thresholds, to some extent, that has to be a subjective judgement by the regulators, and obviously having threshold figures to work with would be an enormous help. More products are being claimed to be free from particular allergens, and at the moment that applies if the particular allergen can't be detected. It would be helpful to have a quantitative measure for allergens that can be applied for foods that want to make those specific claims.

The goals of the FSA are to define levels for the main allergenic foods, below which their accidental presence in the food is deemed not to pose a significant risk at the public health level, and therefore doesn't need to be labelled. Significant risk also needs to be quantified at a public health level. If this can be achieved, then it should lead to consistency among the different retailers and manufacturers over their decisions on when warning statements are used on foods, and this will then increase confidence for the allergic consumer, who will know what the labels mean, what that means in terms of risk for them, and it will help them choose foods more safely.

Working towards achieving these goals, in 2007 the FSA brought together international stakeholders; regulators as well as clinicians and patient groups and food industry from Europe, from America, Canada, Australia and New Zealand to try and look at whether there are methodologies available already that we can use in allergen risk assessment. There are lots of mathematical models that are used in risk assessment for chemicals in food and those methodologies were examined to establish whether they could work and be applied to food allergens. The methodologies were discussed at the workshop, together with their advantages and disadvantages and how such approaches might be taken forward. Information gaps and the research that is needed to take this issue forward were discussed, and this is summarised in a paper that was published at the beginning of 2009, which covers the presentations and the discussion at that workshop (4).

In May 2009 a follow up workshop was held, which centred on defining a tolerable level of risk. Mathematical models can be used to do the risk assessment, but there are obviously some uncertainties in those data, and the safety factors that need to put in to these models to give a level of risk that is tolerable at a population level need to be determined.

Some of the information gaps that were identified established that there isn't a clear picture of the exposure risks for allergic consumers, for example in the UK we have very good information from the national diet and nutrition studies about what non-allergic consumers are eating; the different types of foods, and how much of those foods. It is not known whether those intake data are applicable to the allergic consumer, who may have very different patterns of consumption depending on what allergens they are sensitive to. It is becoming clear from some of the modelling, that the likelihood of an allergic individual eating a type of food, rather than how much of the allergen is present in the food is perhaps one of the key determinants of whether there is a risk of someone having an allergic reaction. So for example, if milk allergic people don't eat plain chocolate, then the milk contamination in the chocolate is not a risk because it's not being consumed. Understanding what governs the choices of allergic consumers and trying to get a better idea of what foods they are actually eating is key. Another factor that needs to be included in the modelling is the variability between different individuals. We know that there is a lot of variability between people in terms of their sensitivity, but also in the same individual there can be a quite significant degree of variation in the sensitivity to an allergen on different occasions. There are a number of external factors that can affect the severity of a reaction, for example if someone has exercised and consumes the allergen to which they are sensitive, they may have a more severe reaction. If they are asthmatic, and their asthma is poorly controlled, their reaction may be more severe on those occasions. Research is needed to try and understand the safety factors that we need to put into the models to allow for this variation, both between people, and within people on different occasions.

The aim of setting the tolerable level of risk for allergens is actually to improve the quality of life for the allergic consumer, because it's clear from a lot of consumer research that it is the fear of having a reaction that is having the most significant effect on the quality of life of the allergic consumer. So if they can have more confidence in the labelling on the foods they are choosing, then this will have a significant impact on their quality of life.

In translating the clinical thresholds for allergens in a few individuals to the management levels for allergens in food, one of the issues to be considered is whether those people that are challenged are really representative of the consumers allergic to that particular food. It might be that the most sensitive people decide that they don't want to be challenged so are excluded, but it could be that the more sensitive people are those that go to the clinics, and they are the subjects chosen for challenges, inferring that a lot of the less sensitive people never get to those clinics, making it difficult to know where the people being challenged actually sit in the spectrum of sensitivity. Therefore, the safety factors that should be applied must be carefully considered.

At the workshop held in May 2009, different stakeholders including consumer organisations, clinicians, as well as industry and regulators met to try and come to a consensus on what is a tolerable level of risk from all their different perspectives, and to think about the individual consumer, as well as at the public health level. The fundamental question 'what are we protecting against' needs to be answered; obviously, management thresholds should aim to protect against severe anaphylactic reactions, but should they also be set at levels to prevent all the mild subjective reactions, such as a small amount of rash or lip tingling? Is it actually feasible to try and protect everybody against all the mild symptoms? Ideally management thresholds would be set at levels that would protect everyone with food allergy, but what proportion of the population is it feasible to protect? There was consensus at the 2009 workshop that zero risk does not exist; a minimal level of risk that is going to be tolerable to people should be the goal of this work.

1.7 Analysing for Allergens

When food incidents related to food allergens are reported, there are occasionally discrepancies between the analytical results for the allergen between what the food business has detected, and the results of testing by the enforcement authority. It may be that different kits are measuring different allergens, or that different kits work better in some food matrices than others. There are certainly issues surrounding the reproducibility of the analytical methods. Very frequently results are reported to the FSA from public analysts and local authorities as 'the allergen is present' or the 'the allergen is there above 25 ppm', rather than giving a quantitative result above 25 ppm. Some of the allergen test kits are quantifiable within certain ranges, and above that range the result is reported as above, making it impossible to know whether 'above 25' means 27 or 250 or more, and so the level of risk is very difficult to judge. Work needs to be done in improving the quantification of analytical methods and to develop robust analytical methods that are sensitive and specific for all the major food allergens. Ideally these methods would also be rapid, and suitable for use by the food industry in their processing and checking. The methods need to be validated using standard reference materials, which are recognised internationally and currently these do not exist. So there is another whole programme of work in this area that still needs to be taken forward.

1.8 References

1. *Guidance on Allergen Management and Consumer Information*, Food Standards Agency, London, England, 2006.

2. *Allergy, What to consider when labelling food – a guide for small business that make or sell prepacked food*, Food Standards Agency, London, England, 2006, reprinted in 2009.

3. food.gov.uk/allergytraining

4. Madsen C. B., Hattersley S., Buck J., Gendel S. M., Houben G. F., Hourihane J. O'B, Mackie A., Mills E.N.C., Nørhede P., Taylor S.L., Crevel R.W.R. Approaches to risk assessment in food allergy: Report from a workshop "developing a framework for assessing the risk from allergenic foods". *Food and Chemical Toxicology*, 2009, 47, 480-9.

2. ALLERGEN MANAGEMENT - ACCIDENTAL TO ACRIMONIOUS: ALLERGY RECALLS AND CONTAMINATION ISSUES

Tony Hines MBE,
Head of Knowledge Transfer and Crisis Management Manager
Leatherhead Food Research

2.1 Introduction

Leatherhead Food Research began to plan a national conference on Food Chain Allergen Management at the beginning of 2009, and the event was to include a presentation entitled 'Allergen Management - Accidental to Acrimonious', which covers some of the issues that were relevant to the allergic community at that time. To provide a focus for the presentation, an acronym was developed for considering food chain allergen management and the responsibility of food and drink manufacturers, retailers, consumers and the Regulatory Authorities:

RECALL
Responsibility for
Effective
Control of
Allergens in
Labelling to limit your
Liability

In summary, food manufacturers need effective control of food allergens with correct labelling declarations and an understanding of their liability under EU Law.

2.2 Food Allergy Research

There was tremendous excitement around the research from Addenbrooke's Hospital in Cambridge following the publication of results of the world's first successful peanut desensitisation programme in February 2009 (1). The work has changed the lives of the children involved in the research, but also raises the possibility that the food and drink industry may become complacent about allergen management. The time frames relating to the methodology behind positive results of clinical research projects such as that done at Addenbrookes being transferred to treatment therapies available in the wider community are long, and it may be five or ten years before this research can make a big difference to the lives of those within the allergic community. However, the positive results of the Addenbrookes research was very exciting news, and listening to, and watching the children that took part in the programme, their parents and other parents at the Anaphylaxis Campaign Annual General Meeting in London on 19th May 2009, it was very interesting to listen to real consumers talking about the real issues that face them and their families. The real life experience of allergic consumers provides the food industry with focus on this issue, and communication to this unique population group, the time frames for research into allergy, and ultimately an allergen-free world, are all very important to them.

2.3 Media Coverage of Food Scares

In early 2009 peanuts seemed to be a constant feature in the news. In the United States The Peanut Corporation of America was involved in one of the largest product recalls in the USA. Salmonella contamination was linked to nine deaths and over 600 reported cases of food poisoning in peanut butter products. Whilst this isn't particularly linked to food allergy, it puts things in perspective, and highlights the vulnerability of the food industry anywhere in the world. On the 14th March 2009 President Obama noted the troubling trend that's seen the average number of outbreaks from contaminated produce and other foods grow to nearly 350 per year - up from 100 per year in the early 1990's.

In crisis management, perspective is very important and I often ask this question: 'What was the most devastating food poisoning incident in modern European History'? The answer - the Spanish Toxic Oil Syndrome of 1981. Leatherhead Food Research did a lot of work on this issue (2). 1000 people died and 25,000 people were seriously injured or permanently disabled. This incident is a measure of why we have systems in place now to protect consumers, whether it is from pathogenic microorganisms, or contamination with non-approved substances.

Figure 2.1 depicts that allergen management and product recalls are often described as 'the journey from hell to sheer hell'. It is a journey often travelled by food manufacturers when they are faced with a product recall; just as things cannot get any worse, they do. The Anaphylaxis Campaign AGM in 2009 demonstrated the difficulties of living with food allergy very clearly, with contributions from consumers who are facing allergy issues. Their journey, for example a family holiday starting on an aeroplane, is often a journey 'from hell to sheer hell' as they try to cope with allergen issues and cross-contamination.

HELL
SHEER HELL
CALAHAN
"Just when I thought things couldn't get any worse!"

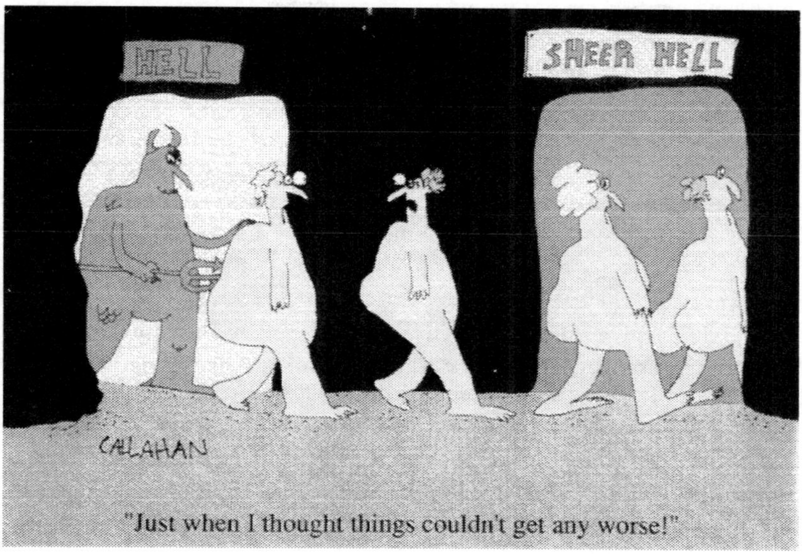

Fig. 2.1. 'hell to sheer hell'

In the early part of 2009 the food industry saw the closure of yet another issue with the publishing of Professor Hugh Pennington's report on the *E.coli* 0157 incident in South Wales in 2005 (3). This was the second public enquiry chaired by Professor Pennington on *E.coli* 0157. This incident is another sad example of a serious food crisis where a young consumer died.

The Belgian dioxin crisis in 1999 is the perfect front page news from a journalist's perspective. The headline said 'FAST FOOD POISON ALERT' and was accompanied by a rural picture of HRH Prince Charles. The second headline 'FOOD CRISIS GRIPS EUROPE' focussed the minds of consumers, demonstrated the vulnerability of the food chain, provided entertainment and presumably increased daily sales. After the dioxin incident, new legislation was introduced and the Rapid Alert System for Food and Feed in Europe was implemented. Often after a crisis the regulatory framework changes, and new legislation is introduced. In 2008 in Ireland there was another dioxin scare which resulted in a massive product recall. This was almost a repeat of the dioxin crisis in Belgium in 1999, and what was concerning, was that on looking at the details of the Irish scare, it was very similar to the one in Belgium, so lessons had not been learned from that previous incident.

Also in 1999, and almost simultaneous with the dioxin scare in Belgium, Coca Cola had a major problem with their products being banned in several European countries due to suspected contamination. It could be argued that their massive product recall was predominantly driven by the media because the crisis involved an American company in Europe who perhaps failed to appreciate the ongoing food industry scare in Belgium. The European media wrote vociferously about Coca Cola and the story remained in the European print media for weeks. The recall apparently cost the company $60 million. However, at a public enquiry into the 'illness' attributed to Coca Cola products, the French Consumer Affairs Minister said that no link had been found between the products and the cases of sickness reported in France. No causal link in a recall driven by the Media! No evidence was found from analytical testing to support a product recall. Interesting as this may seem, the recall still cost Coca Cola $60 million.

The threats and fears from Avian Influenza H5N1 in 2005 and its potential impact on the European flock, egg supply, ingredients from eggs and the food industry's ability to produce food in a pandemic, gave rise to dramatic headlines. For example 'No turkeys at Christmas', ideally timed at the end of October when consumers see the first Christmas decorations and begin to consider their Christmas lunch. As the festive season approached, turkey farmers breathed a sigh of relief that their annual high income earning period was not going to be incinerated.

The media views the food industry as a source of entertainment, the key point being that negative stories related to food sell newspapers, and newspapers exist to make a profit. The media report negative food-related events, and sadly the food industry has lots of negative events.

2.4 Acrimonious or Malicious Contamination

The use of the word 'acrimonious' at the beginning of this piece is quite emotive - why is it appropriate in this context? 15 years' experience in crisis management has demonstrated that acrimonious contamination is nothing particularly new, and some incidents will be familiar to those who work in the food industry. In 2005 a major UK bakery was subject to a number of incidents relating to glass and needles being added to their products maliciously. Security at the factory was increased significantly to prevent further sabotage of their products. The recall of Findus Crispy Pancakes in 1999 due to malicious contamination with glass involved a number of products and ended with a court case to prosecute the factory worker implicated in the contamination. To the company and its staff it was fairly obvious who had contaminated the products with 'small cubic pieces of glass', but when the case got to court there was insufficient evidence to secure a prosecution. So acrimonious contamination, or deliberate intentional contamination, within a food factory environment is not new.

2.5 Product Recall

Tracking the layout, design and placement of product recall notices in newspapers in the UK over a number of years shows an interesting history of the type of products that have been recalled, the reasons for the recall, and the way that the company concerned has used the media to communicate the recall to the general public.

The first 'product recall notice' that Leatherhead has on record dates back to March 1997, and interestingly it is not headed 'product recall', but 'Important Customer Safety Notice' and relates to chocolate body paint, and appeared in the press just after Valentine's Day, which is a time when chocolate body paint is apparently a very popular present. Following this recall, a risk assessment was conducted by the company who made the body paint, who subsequently recalled a children's Chocolate Spread because the risk associated with this product, which was co-packaged in the same factory in the Netherlands as the chocolate body paint, was seen to be much higher than that associated with the chocolate body paint.

From 2000 onwards, the words Product Recall were used more commonly on these types of alerts. The food industry began to realise and understand the importance of removing defective products from shelves, and the regulatory authorities were demanding that this should happen. Why were they demanding that defective products be removed from sale? A good example is a case where the headline that appeared in the press in July 2000 read 'ALLERGY VICTIM DIES AS LABEL HIDES NUT ALERT'. Food has the capacity occasionally to kill. Sadly these things happen, and reinforce the importance of managing allergenic ingredients, and why products with the wrong ingredients or the wrong packaging should be removed from the shelves and the problem communicated to consumers very quickly.

Product recalls can happen to the very biggest companies, the very smallest companies and everyone in between. Some of the examples the Food Standards Agency (FSA) gives in Chapter 1 highlight the reasons that product recalls are very important. A record of the page numbers on which these product recall notices appear in the newspapers, together with their size shows that their prominence and position in the newspapers vary enormously. Food companies should consider the question: do you have a better due diligence defence when your notice to consumers is published on page 14, rather than on page 57 or page 66, or even in The Sun on page 90?

Figure 2.2 shows a Notice to Allergy Suffers (it was not called a recall) for Chocolate Christmas Tree Decorations. This recall took place in December 2003, and another recall of Milk Chocolate Miniatures Advent Calendars took place in 2005. The connection between the two recalls is that the inner packaging and the outer packaging can contain completely different allergen declarations and messages. There have been a number of systems introduced over many years to try to improve packaging and labelling of foods in order to prevent these situations from arising.

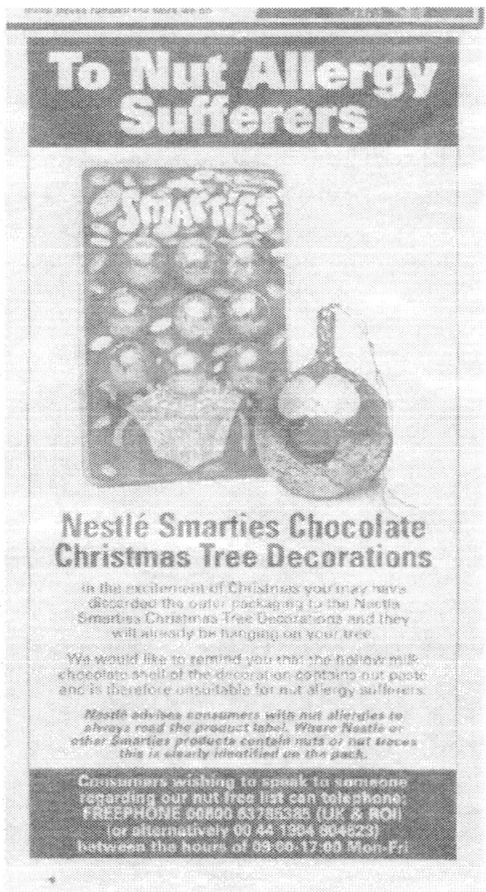

Fig. 2.2. Product recall for chocolate tree decorations

Another example of a product recall for Gravy Granules is dated 1st April 2009. The product was recalled because the wrong type of gravy granules had been put in the packaging, meaning that the product contained milk and egg, which were not mentioned on the label. This wasn't an April Fools' Day joke, but demonstrates that recalls relating to incorrect allergen labelling still happen: the right product is put in the wrong box, or the right box contains the wrong product. The Food Standards Agency believes that systems are improving, but the number of recalls to the end of April in 2009 at least equalled or slightly exceeded the same period in 2008. What is interesting is that 7% of product recalls related to food incidents in 2007, much the same figure as in 2008. Roughly 7% of 1312 incidents, which amounts to 96 incidents, involved the right product being put in the wrong box, or there being insufficient labelling, or ingredients present that haven't been declared on the label correctly.

2.6 Media Coverage of Food Allergy

A media article from 2005, entitled 'PEANUT LOVER'S KISS OF DEATH', relates to a young Canadian girl who, the media reported, died after kissing her boyfriend goodnight. He had apparently eaten a peanut butter sandwich hours earlier. It subsequently became clear that whilst the story attracted a high impact headline it may not reflect a true picture of the incident. This is an example of how far the reach of allergy precautions must extend for anyone with an allergy – particularly in teenagers. As well as counselling them on personal and social development, they also have to contend with the very real hazard of living with a severe food allergy, and must adapt their behaviour in all aspects of daily life accordingly.

In more examples of press headlines: 'GIRL,13 DIES AFTER EATING CHOCOLATE BAR' from 2004, and 'KILLED BY AN ALLERGIC REACTION TO CURRY' from 2005; the vulnerability of allergic people to exposure to allergens is such that it requires every effort that the food industry can possibly give to prevent these events. The first case is a young teenage girl who died at a bus stop apparently after eating a bar of chocolate, although subsequent investigations refute that dairy allergy was the main cause of her death. The second example is of a male who died after eating peanut in a takeaway curry, without his close family being aware of his diagnosed allergy.

2.7 Due Diligence Defence

The food industry needs to understand what a food emergency involves, and must understand what is expected of it as an industry. When talking about the management of food allergens the case of the mouse found in a chocolate bar is an important piece of case law, but why? In this particular case, the chocolate bar manufacturer was cleared of breaking food hygiene law because it could prove that it had taken all reasonable steps to prevent this from happening. This particular case determined that HACCP was a good due diligence defence. 'It shall be a defence for the person charged to prove that he took all reasonable precautions'. In the management of food allergens, the use of HACCP as the management tool is the way forward and is now generally accepted. The case of the 'rodent in a chocolate bar' is a stark reminder to ensure that the food industry learns from this and every other product recall or food issue.

When looking at the global implications of allergen management, whether considering Australia and New Zealand, or indeed anywhere else in the world, the Authorities in other regions are looking to the UK and mainland Europe to see what is being done to manage allergens, and to protect vulnerable consumers.

Within the European Regulatory Framework there is an immediate duty to recall potentially harmful products, especially those containing undeclared allergens, and to pass this information to the Authorities and consumers. There are traditional and emerging channels of communication to achieve this; the traditional means including the print media, in-store notices and web sites. Emerging channels include till receipts, text messaging, customer loyalty cards, social networking sites, or through the various consumer bodies direct to their Members, for example the Anaphylaxis Campaign and Allergy UK.

The triggers for a crisis are well-known and can be found in figure 2.3; they materialise with a degree of regularity. The focus here is on illness caused by allergenic ingredients, but there are lots more reasons for a food recall, and faulty packaging or faulty labelling are just part of that story. Accidental contamination does occasionally occur, and triggers a product recall.

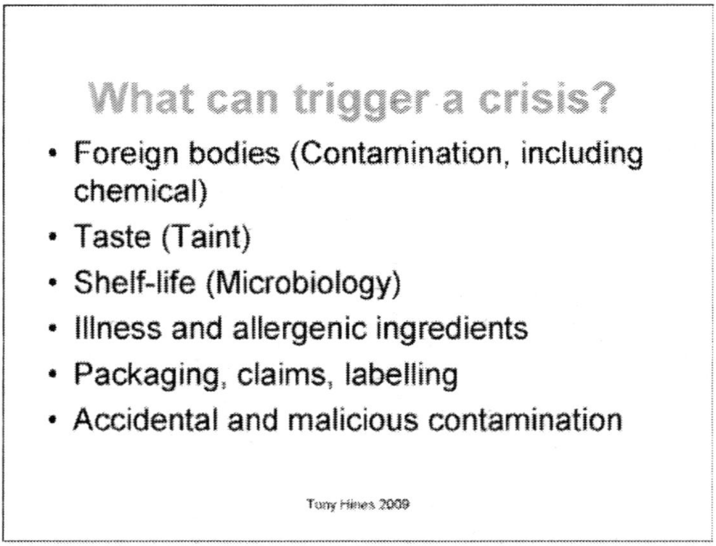

Fig. 2.3. Causes of a food crisis

Under the wider regulatory framework, there is a responsibility to be able to trace products, to know where products are, and to remove them from sale as quickly as possible. There are a number of assessment models available to make the decision on whether to recall a product, of which a threat rating is one. Figure

2.4 illustrates a threat rating matrix. To illustrate the parameters, the ratings range from discomfort, to fatality, and when the level of threat surrounding allergenic ingredients rises to a point where there is the potential for fatalities, the products have to be recalled immediately. A major consideration is where the products in question are in the distribution chain. If they are still under the manufacturer's or retailer's control, on pallets in the factory – a crisis that would generally rate a high score (64-80), in this situation has a low score (1-3) providing that the product is retained, the manufacturer or retailer ensures its security, and it is not released into the market place. There have been plenty of examples within the food industry where a batch of product is being held safe and secure, and a colleague, unaware of why the product is 'isolated', releases it out into the distribution chain. Human error is often the causative agent of a wider recall.

Risk / Threat Assessment Model for Decision Making
An aid to help you assess the impact of an incident

Threat Rating Matrix

SEVERITY	LIKELIHOOD → very unlikely	unlikely	possible	likely	very likely	
Discomfort	1	2	3	4	5	minor
	2	4	6	8	10	appreciable
	4	8	12	16	20	major
	8	16	24	32	40	severe
Death	16	32	48	64	80	catastrophic

Tony Hines 2009

Fig. 2.4. Risk/Threat Assessment Model

Figure 2.5 depicts a product recall notice for ground paprika that is not effective in its purpose of communicating a problem with a product to the public. The notice only measures 7.3 by 5 cm, and this example gives fuel to the argument for having legislation ensuring that product recall notices are a certain size and within the first 10 pages of a newspaper, as is the case in some other parts of the world.

Compare it with the image in figure 2.2, for Chocolate Christmas Tree Decorations, published in December 2003, that appeared in at least eight different daily papers with an average size of 15cm x 25cm. There are significant differences in the cost of these notices, and different approaches to public relations but in the case of the notice for ground paprika, the manufacturer was not communicating very effectively with its consumers, and this begs the question: 'where is the due diligence defence'?

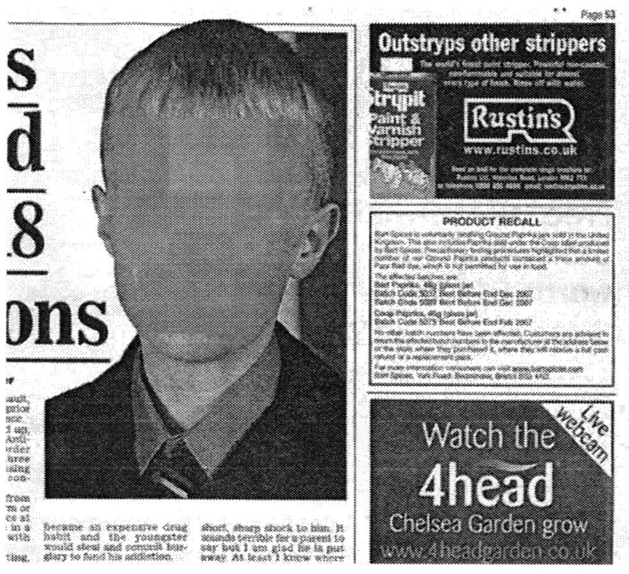

Fig. 2.5. Example of an inadequate product recall notice

2.8 Product Recall Insurance

Product Recall Insurance is available to food companies, and in order to negotiate the best terms for insurance, a number of insurance companies were canvassed as to the management systems that need to be in place. All the companies questioned stated that a food producer's HACCP management and product management systems need to be better than exceptionally good, in order to negotiate better terms. There must be recall plans, mock recalls conducted, training, crisis management planning, and accurate traceability. All food companies should have these in place as a minimum, but insurance companies require an extra level of planning in place in the event of a recall. This could be implementation of the Anaphylaxis Campaign or BRC Standard. Accidental and malicious contamination within a factory is covered by some companies (see figure 2.6). Other companies will go through a risk assessment process, and identify how consumers could be harmed by your products, so therefore the number of allergenic ingredients used on site becomes an issue. To be considered as a new client a food manufacturer will have to have exceptional quality systems, great crisis management training, excellent traceability systems, independent audits and - this is the critical bit - an adherence to Standards is a significant benefit.

Trigger - Accidental Contamination, Malicious Contamination and Extortion

Coverage is provided for:

- Pre-Recall Expenses
- Recall Expenses
- Third Party Recall Expenses
- Loss of Gross Profit
- Rehabilitation
- Increased Cost of Working
- Extortion Demands

Fig. 2.6. Insurance coverage for accidental and malicious contamination, and extortion

2.9 Malicious Contamination with Peanuts

In February 2009 reports of a court case became public in which the headline read: 'NUT FREE FACTORY 'NUKED' BY STRAY PEANUTS'. This particular case sparked the use of the word 'acrimonious' for this chapter, and involved the deliberate contamination of a sausage production factory with peanuts. It is true that as much panic, with a massive cost, can be caused by throwing a few handfuls of peanuts around a factory as can be triggered by threatening to contaminate foods with chemical or biological agents. This particular case was a new incident because it involved contamination with peanuts, whereas the cases described previously involved contamination with glass. This is a serious message to the whole food industry, especially taking into account the cost of £1.2 million associated with cleaning up the factory. This incident led to a court case twice and was eventually dismissed through insufficient evidence. The accused was acquitted; however if the accused didn't do it someone else did. The company concerned has issued a report to the Anaphylaxis Campaign about the increased security measures that they have introduced in the factory. The food industry needs to be aware of who is working in their factories, and the threats that individuals may pose.

More examples of intentional contamination, either in the factory, distribution or retail environments, include a threat to poison biscuits and deliberate contamination of bread with foreign objects. It is often reported that sacking agency and other workers is generally considered to be a trigger for factory contamination.

Within most food factories, general and allergen management needs to focus more on people issues. Take the issue of putting the right product in the wrong packaging, malicious contamination can and does happen, and there should be systems and structures in place to make food production work smoothly. However, people make systems happen, and people need to work in the right culture. People need good management, they need great leadership, and they need clarity of communication to understand why they or the equipment mustn't put the right product in the wrong box, and the 'big picture' implications of doing it. People need commitment from management, and people enjoy an 'eyes-wide-open policy'.

To prevent a product recall early intervention is required. There is an analogy with the early diagnosis of a chronic illness; the successful management of a chronic illness requires early diagnosis, and if we look at the statistics, around 50% of food product recalls in the UK and the US are because there was the right product in the wrong box. If this is transposed into a factory setting, early diagnosis and intervention are essential. The eyes-wide-open policy is a tremendous step towards preventing the right product being put into the wrong box. Everyone in the factory should be encouraged to become an auditor, a gate keeper, an inspector, or a policeman so that prevalence of errors may reduce. Early diagnosis may just stop mislabelled products leaving the factory and therefore may prevent a recall.

To conclude, Food Chain Allergen Management is not just about labelling, it is about all embracing GMP and HACCP. It's about common sense all the time, everywhere and involving everybody in the factory. It's about time management, it's about language, it's about training, it's about appreciation of the issues and it's always obvious afterwards!

1. http://www.cuh.org.uk/addenbrookes/news/2009/feb/peanut_allergy.html

2. Kochhar S.P., Rossell J.B. The Spanish toxic oil syndrome, Nutrition and Food Science. 1984, (90), 14-15.

3. http://wales.gov.uk/splash;jsessionid=QbphKJ0Q1gS8Y1QtCgbzM1svjHY9GYTQJYyRCsY3HmTn6dYhkyTF!-1386067949?orig=/ecolidocs/3008707/reporten.pdf

3. ANAPHYLAXIS CAMPAIGN STANDARD

Neil Griffiths BSc Hons.,MChemA.,CChem.,CSci.,FRSC.,FIFST.,FSOFHT
Neil Griffiths Consultants

3.1 Introduction

This chapter will provide background to the generation of what is an important standard by the Anaphylaxis Campaign. The Standard, which is an extremely useful best practice document for the food industry will be addressed in some detail, including its certification scheme and a logo.

3.2 The Anaphylaxis Campaign Standard

The Anaphylaxis Campaign first raised the subject of a Standard for the food industry in 2003. As an organisation, the Anaphylaxis Campaign has a deeper level of understanding, because the majority of Campaign staff either have family members, or they themselves suffer from food allergy. The Campaign is being proactive in trying to do something about allergen management in food production, and going about it in a different way, by actually engaging the industry and talking to the industry about it. The initiative to create the Standard was started around the time of tremendously rapid changes in allergen labelling law, which has been a challenge for the food industry to catch up with.

The Anaphylaxis Campaign initiated discussion to create an industry Standard born from the views of genuine food allergic members. The concept began with the establishment of what best practice is. At this stage, the Food Standards Agency hadn't yet produced its own Guidance, and was willing to provide some financial support to the Anaphylaxis Campaign to move forward in the developing of this Standard.

3.3 Food Allergen Legislation

There is no single piece of legislation covering food allergens; there is both criminal and civil law, and obviously, there is a lot of concern within the industry about the liability in this area. The food industry is aware of both the criminal law involved in relation to labelling, in particular where a fine and imprisonment can be imposed, and the civil element in relationship to damages. In the development of these Directives, obviously the main one is the primary food labelling Directive, but the important one that started to introduce the requirements to list these major allergens within the ingredients list (the ones that have been positively added) came in 2003. Amendments are now underway to add other allergens. Directive 2006/13/EC introduced the requirement for labelling Lupin and Molluscs, together with Directive 2007/68/EC, which concerns the derivatives and the exemptions and derogations. Following the European Food Safety Authority assessment of those, there was clarification on which derivatives need to be labelled, and which ones are exempt from labelling. The amendment of Directive 2000/13/EC contains all the allergen labelling requirements including lupins, molluscs, gastropods, bivalves or cephalopods and products thereof.

The Food Labelling (Declaration of Allergens) (England) Regulations 2007 obviously implemented the changes in the Directive into UK law. The transition period lasted until 23 December 2008; if a product was marked and labelled before that date and it didn't meet the requirements to include lupin and mollusc on the label, then it is still legal.

Temporarily exempted derivatives listed in Table 3.I have NOT been granted permanent status and will, therefore, have to be ingredient listed with an indication of their allergenic origin.

TABLE 3.I
Temporarily exempted derivatives that have not been granted permanent status

Allergen	Derivative
Eggs	Lysozyme (produced from egg) used in wine Egg albumin fining agent for wine and cider
Fish	Fish gelatin or Isinglass fining agent for cider
Milk	Milk (casein) fining agent, wine and cider
Nuts	Nuts (Almonds/walnuts) used as flavour in spirits
Celery	Celery leaf and seed oil, Celery seed oleoresin
Mustard	Mustard oil and mustard seed oil, Mustard seed oleoresin

3.4 Liability

Clearly, liability can occur when an allergen is present in a product, which should have been labelled as containing the allergen. The presence of the allergen in the food may be due to deliberate addition where the allergen should definitely be mentioned in the labelling, or it may be due to its presence as a contaminant. Clearly the situation can arise, where there is an allergen in a product that has been incorrectly labelled, or even a mix up of the labelling between the allergen-containing product and a similar product that does not contain a particular allergen. Primarily there is a very great concern about the potential impact on brands of getting allergen labelling wrong and a recent survey by Reading Scientific Services showed that of the product recalls initiated, over 50% are now down to allergens, and in the United States this figure is closer to 60%. The commercial cost of a recall is considerable, both in terms of the recall itself, but also in brand damage, which is harder to quantify.

The use of “may contain” or similar labelling is widespread, and it could be argued that may contain labelling is used by some companies as an easy way out; a means of not necessarily introducing the best practices that will reduce the risk to a minimum within the business. It is becoming very, very difficult for those who suffer from anaphylaxis to be able to evaluate risk, and make informed decisions about the food they eat, because when there are so many warning labels being used, there is a tendency for consumers to ignore them.

The presence of allergens as risk factors in products should be put into context in terms of other elements of risk for food producers. The food industry manages risk for contaminants on a daily basis; that might be a microbiological contaminant, or a chemical contaminant or a physical contaminant. What food businesses are doing is reducing those risks as much as they can through the adoption of best practice to achieve a level of risk that is at a minimum which that particular company can support commercially. Food businesses live with this risk every day, so why is it that ‘may contain’ labelling appears on so many products?

If best practices are put in place to reduce the risk of inadvertent contamination of allergens to a minimum, there is no difference between that, and doing the same in a microbiological context and not labelling your product with “may contain *Listeria*” or “pathogens” on products. Why are allergens perceived to be a much greater liability? *Salmonella* and *Listeria* in foods can cause fatalities when eaten as easily as allergens. It could be that stating ‘may contain nuts’ on your product restricts sales of your products to a relatively small number of people, whereas if the statement ‘may contain Salmonella’ was used, marketing the product at all would be futile.

There are defences in criminal law in this area, and to avoid the potential of prosecution operation of a due diligence defence is important here within the United Kingdom. In any civil case against the industry, of which there are very few here in the UK, courts will assess whether everything reasonable has been done to try and make sure that a problem such as microbiological or allergen contamination hasn’t occurred, in establishing damages. The operation of best practice is well understood; the key issue is how many companies have best practice documents sitting on shelves unused and are not actually introducing them into their factories, and making sure that they are working. Having a working best practice policy is clearly the important element in relationship to a due diligence defence.

3.5 The Need for Standards

There are some extremely good standards available, notably, the British Retail Consortium (BRC) Food Safety Standard. However, there are times when an issue arises in the food industry which requires a level of concentration that it is not possible to provide in the generality of the food safety system. Indeed there may be a negative impact on that food safety system if an evaluator has to go into a business and try and devote the concentration that is needed into this new area of food safety. This may bias the assessor against their overall task of trying to implement the overall food safety standard. It is not unusual for the food industry on occasion to have areas of food safety for which it needs to devote more attention. Now is a time that allergens require a level of concentration that can't necessarily be delivered within the generality of the best practice systems for food that are currently in place. In the future, general best practice systems should be able to incorporate allergens, but for the moment, the handling of allergens requires specific, detailed attention. This view was mirrored by the United Kingdom Accreditation Service (UKAS) when pilot trials on the Anaphylaxis Campaign Standard were run to set up certification schemes within factories. The UKAS view was that it is almost impossible for an evaluator to apply the required level of concentration on allergens without extending the timescale of evaluations quite substantially. In essence, allergens currently require a separate audit.

3.6 Allergen Management Standards

Some standards include allergen requirements - some at a basic level; some standards are not designed to address the labelling issues. Auditors are not necessarily trained in allergen requirements, and The Anaphylaxis Campaign has struggled to find evaluators trained in this area. There are difficulties involved in bolting on new elements to existing standards, and schemes. Independence is particularly important, particularly in a circumstance where trust is needed to be engendered in the consumer.

3.6.1 The Anaphylaxis Campaign Standard

The Anaphylaxis Campaign is the owner of its new Standard, and of the certification scheme that accompanies it. The Anaphylaxis Campaign Standards were generated with the collaboration of Bodycote Health Sciences, and Dorothy Cullinane, who previously worked in the allergen area for Sainsbury's. The Food Standards Agency provided a grant to support development of the Standard. The process is outlined in Table 3.II and involved a significant consultation exercise including 3 major consultation meetings on the Standard, and a postal consultation with all those people who wanted to be involved, which provided a very strong representative group of stakeholders. Most of the critical stages in Table 3.II have been accomplished. As well as a manufacturing standard, a Standard has been created on catering, which is currently with the FSA for evaluation.

TABLE 3.II
Critical Stages in the development of the Anaphylaxis Campaign Standard

- Draft Manufacturing and Catering standard produced
- UKAS became involved
- Wider consultation held
- Guidance on the Manufacturing Standard produced and Manufacturing Standard revised.
- Agreement achieved on final Manufacturing Standard and Guidance with formal recognition by UKAS
- Copies of Manufacturing standard made available for purchase through Highfield Publications.
- Catering Standard revised and Catering Guidance document generated.
- Training Course Generated and launched
- Recognition sought by UKAS of Catering Standard and Guidance
- Certification bodies can seek accreditation by UKAS
- Evaluations to the Manufacturing and Catering Standards can start

The aim of the Standard is the reduction of risk through the management of allergens throughout the whole supply chain. The general food law regulation with its “one back one forward” approach in relation to traceability, would not in my view be sufficient to run a due diligence defence here in the United Kingdom. Legally, food companies have got to go further than the general food law regulation, which merely establishes a baseline.

What the Anaphylaxis Campaign Standard has been created to do is to enable increased confidence in the supply chain, and to communicate risk to consumers. The Anaphylaxis Campaign Standard is in place so that companies achieving the certification are seen to produce products at a lower risk of allergen contamination, and are able to meet a due diligence challenge. The scope of the Standard covers ingredients labelled as is legally required, and has been limited to the allergens legally laid down within the labelling Directive. The Standard could be applied to other allergens; however the scope for the certification is the allergens contained within the labelling regulations. The Standard covers allergen advice boxes, and may contain labelling.

3.6.2 Allergen thresholds and the declaration of free-from

Free from products are not part of the Standard because of the issue of thresholds. When the Standard was in development, the original requirement was to create an add-on module to the Standard to cover free-from, and the view from UKAS (who would be required to shoulder some liability associated with the Standard if it was going to become part of certification) was that to certify products free-from allergens without established allergen thresholds was too great a liability. This is noteworthy not least because there are a lot of companies who are currently producing free-from product ranges. But the truth of the matter is that we couldn't get free-from involved in the certification scheme. There is a new Regulation (Commission Regulation (41/2009 20th Jan)) on foods suitable for people intolerant to gluten, which requires that the Anaphylaxis Campaign Standard be modified. This is because this Regulation imposes for the first time, a limit of 20 ppm, or 20 milligram per kilo for gluten, for a gluten-free claim in both a PARNUT food and a normal food and a 100 milligram per kilo limit for gluten in a PARNUT food for a very low gluten claim. This is one of the first regulations to establish a threshold, and the Standard has had to be modified to allow a free-from gluten claim, because the regulations allow it. Incorporating free-from limits for any other allergens is on hold until thresholds are developed in that regard.

The contents of the Standard cover risk, management, environment, labelling and communication, and the Standard, as well as the guidelines to go with it have been developed in the same way. A Standard and Guidelines have also been developed for catering, but have not yet been published. The different phases and sections of the Standard are depicted in Figure 3.1.

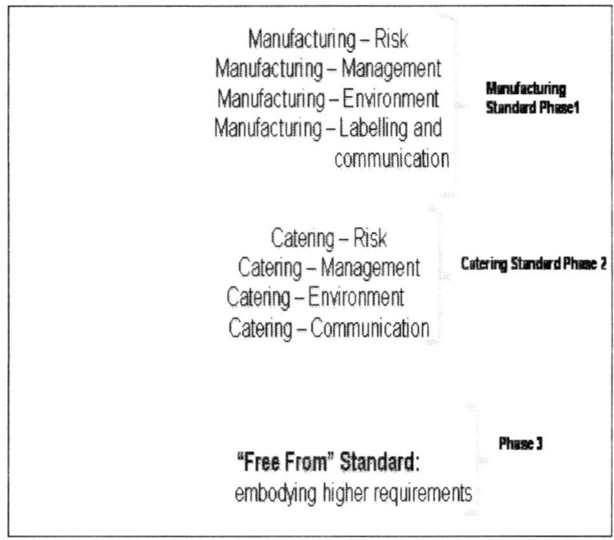

Fig. 3.1. Phases and composition of the Anaphylaxis Campaign Standard

The key areas addressed within the Standard are Training; Allergen Policy; Management; Risk Assessment; Preventing Cross Contamination; Crisis Management; Supplier Assurance; Factory Procedures and Environment, including transport, storage, segregation, scheduling, waste management, cleaning and emergency action; Labelling and communication; Personnel and management review. It is a very comprehensive standard, and the difference between this standard and guidance is that:

1) it can be evaluated or audited against
2) it mirrors the systems and procedures that the food industry already uses for other contaminants.

One might question why the industry needs another standard, when there is guidance on allergens available. Standards enable the proper procedures to be put in place by suppliers, so that should manufacturers assess their suppliers, there is a benchmark against which to measure their allergen management.

One of the important findings that came out of the consultation was the massive need within the industry for training in allergen management at the moment. Before best practice can be implemented, there needs to be the understanding within the businesses what that best practice is. There is a compulsory requirement in the Standard that at least one person within the organisation that the Anaphylaxis Campaign is going to certify should have a detailed understanding of the systems and procedures necessary to implement the allergen management systems and procedures laid out in the Standard. A training course has been devised through consultation. This has been through several revision phases following pilot trials, and runs primarily over two days providing training on all of the areas covered by the Standard.

The Anaphylaxis Campaign Standard is very closely linked to HACCP, and the reason for structuring the Standard in that way is because food businesses are already familiar with HACCP principles. There is a clear structure within the Standard, and the concept of pre-requisite programmes contained in it are compatible with those for food hygiene. There is a school of thought that HACCP ought not to be applied in this particular area as: it is not an appropriate tool; there isn't a critical control point in allergen contact because it cannot be controlled; it is difficult to establish critical limits; allergens can't be controlled by temperature, and allergens cannot be cleaned with disinfectants, biocides and the cleaning process, but control relies on physical removal. A means around this argument is to eliminate the hazard through pre-requisite programmes if it can't be controlled. This doesn't remove the requirement for checking, validating and testing, and it does not take away the concept of critical limits.

The components of a ten step plan that can be used in order to generate a logical allergen management plan are laid out in figure 3.2, and the plan is part of the Anaphylaxis Campaign training course.

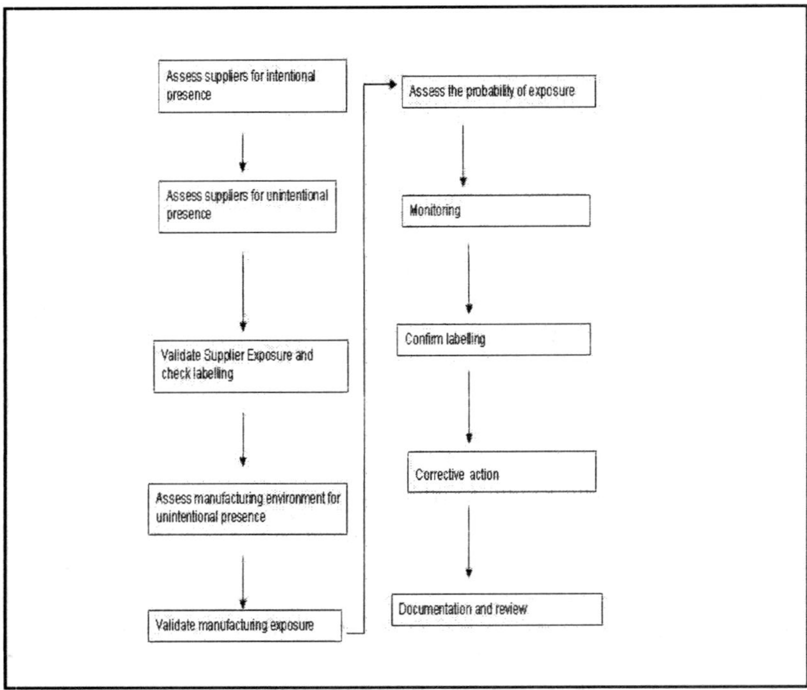

Fig. 3.2. Ten steps required in an allergen management programme

3.7 Testing for Allergens

Manufacturers of test kits for detecting and determining the presence of allergens provide information on the performance criteria of the methodologies that are available for allergen testing. In many instances the testing kits available are not sensitive enough to do the job that the food industry requires of them. Development of more accurate testing kits for allergens needs to be undertaken in tandem with research into allergen thresholds. It may be possible to achieve accurate results within laboratories, but it is difficult to obtain the same results for allergen analyses between laboratories. That is important from a UK law perspective because the law works on a formal sampling approach, and a formal sample must be able to be divided in 3 parts and for 3 laboratories to achieve the same analytical result; otherwise it should not be used in a court room. It's a fantastic opportunity for those involved in testing, but there is a tremendous challenge involved in it as well.

As part of the training course associated with the Anaphylaxis Campaign Standard, testing companies provide information to help explain how to take samples, what to sample, and when to sample. It is important to understand in more detail what testing is available; is DNA testing relevant, how the results are interpreted, what action should be taken, and how much confidence can be placed in the testing. Other factors to consider are listed in Table 3.III.

TABLE 3.III
Risk factors in allergen assessment

1. Level of allergen required to provoke a reaction
2. Prevalence of allergy in the population
3. How allergenic is the material
4. Any target groups?
5. Physical nature of the allergen?
6. Type of production environment

Best practice for allergens has now been established. Should best practice be applied to a certification model? Third party certification is necessary in order to: introduce consistency into the allergen management control system; to avoid suppliers undergoing multiple audits by different retailers; to avoid misunderstanding of legal requirements, or conflicting or unrealistic expectations.

Without proper certification, the duplication costs to the industry can be significant.

Best practice advice in this area currently include:

1. The Anaphylaxis Campaign Standards and Guidelines to Increase Trust and Information about Allergens in Food: Food manufacturing and Catering
2. FSA best Practice Guidance on Managing Food Allergens with Particular Reference to Avoiding Cross-Contamination and Using Appropriate Advisory Labelling
3. BRC Global Standard for Food Safety Issue 5

The Anaphylaxis Campaign certification scheme is based on product certification, which is different to a management certification scheme.

The Anaphylaxis Campaign conducted a survey among its members, and asked whether they would like the Campaign to communicate to them the names of those companies that are demonstrating they are doing the best job that they possibly can by operating the Campaign's Standard, and being certified under the Standard, and the answer was not surprisingly, an unequivocal yes. Allergic consumers have difficulty knowing which companies to trust in terms of producing food that is safe for them to eat, and would like to be supplied with information to show them which companies are going the extra distance to manage allergens in their production facility. In order to demonstrate publicly which companies are following the Anaphylaxis Campaign Standard, this logo was designed to accompany the scheme.

Fig. 3.3. Anaphylaxis Campaign certification scheme logo

The reasons for using a logo to identify users of the scheme are because consumers want to know which products met the requirements, but the logo is not a general sign of approval for people affected by different allergens. The logo is a signpost rather than an endorsement because there are liability issues to consider in this context. The logo should be used within an allergen information box or adjacent to an ingredients list.

The use of a standard of this sort can go a long way in reducing the risk of communicating the wrong allergen information, but cannot eliminate the risk entirely. It is important that this concept is communicated to customers; it is not appropriate to give cast iron guarantees of freedom from a specific allergen based on this certification.

4. CONTROLLING AND COMMUNICATING

Dr Geoff Spriegel
Director of Global Standards and Technical Services
British Retail Consortium

4.1 Introduction

Management of allergens is a major issue. Cases of anaphylactic shock from food reported in the media demonstrate that the food industry still has a way to go in completely controlling food allergens.

When the BRC Global Standard for Food Safety was first created some 10 years ago, it focussed on hygiene and foreign body control because these were the issues that were prevalent at the time. When allergen management first became an issue of note, it was regarded by a lot of the industry as a significant problem for a very small proportion of consumers. Clearly over the last decade it has become accepted that more people are allergic to different foods than was originally thought and the incidence and severity of allergic reactions are becoming more prominent. As a consequence there are more product recalls related to allergens than used to be the case. If the food industry is going to address this, it will have to manage allergens better than it has done previously, and the detail of allergen management will receive greater attention.

4.2 The BRC Standard

The BRC is constantly improving the infrastructure for BRC third party certification, as its uptake expands across the world. Greater resources are now in place with the capability to make significant enhancements to compliance with the scheme. That investment in resources has been supported by investment in technology, including a new interactive web site and directory.

The BRC operate a range of Global Schemes, with 14,000 certificated sites across the world. It is inevitable that as uptake increases across the world The Schemes become more difficult to manage. Various checks and balances are being introduced to enhance control. BRC don't themselves carry out audits; there is a network of certification bodies to carry out this work. There are about 100 certification bodies conducting audits against the Food Standard alone. The BRC is monitoring certification bodies and the way they manage and train their auditors. In addition to the wide network of certification bodies a large group of between 60 and 70 approved training providers, who can deliver training against the BRC Standards in the local language of their country has been developed. The BRC international network of training providers, certification bodies and certificated sites, now probably extends to about 90 countries.

Issue 5 of the Food Standard was published following feedback from a wide range of stakeholders. A working group was established, consisting of about 30 experts from retailers, food manufacturers, and certification bodies. The Standard was edited throughout 2007 and was distributed for international consultation; comments were received from about 250 parties across the world. As part of this work, the FSA data of product recalls for the previous 3 years were reviewed to ensure the latest food safety issues were considered. The Standard was published in January 2008 with an effective date of 1 July 2008, and audits against the standard are now being conducted.

What are the key points of improvement? Experience within both food manufacture and retailing shows that any food safety system is only going to be effective with Senior Management Commitment. One goal of the BRC Standard was to make the requirements for Management Commitment and HACCP more auditable than they have been in the past. Other areas that were considered to be important were Customer Review and Customer Focus; there is now a requirement that companies develop closer relationships with their customers. Product Design and Development were also included, which previously weren't part of the Standard. More stringent requirements for labelling control, including packaging on the line were also introduced, because clearly one of the issues that have been identified as far as allergens are concerned is getting the right product consistently in the right packaging.

There was also feedback that improvement to the requirements for allergen management should be considered. This created much debate with the rewrite group because some parties thought that greater detail on cleaning was needed in the Standard, other people were of the opinion that glass control needed greater detail. In producing a management Standard it is essential that individual items are viewed within the context of the overall Standard. The section on allergen management was improved quite considerably, but within the context of a general Food Safety Standard – all sections must carry appropriate weight.

4.3 Allergen Coverage in the BRC Standard

To raise the profile for the handling of allergens the decision was taken to make allergen control a fundamental requirement of the BRC Standard, and to cover the areas listed below:

- Allergens to be listed within raw materials
- Identify routes of contamination with prescriptive areas to consider – physical or time segregation, dedicated equipment, food brought on site
- Validation of claims made
- Validation of cleaning and waste control
- Emphasis on training and management review

4.4 Inter-country differences

The Standard has been translated into 13 different languages. In each case the translation is an exact copy of the English Version but the North American translation is a good example of the problems encountered in managing allergens in different countries, and the differences in the legislation in the countries in which the products are made available for sale.

The BRC standard is gaining increasing application in the United States at the moment; it is the area of the world where use of the Standard is growing the fastest. A Technical Advisory Committee has been formed in the States, and one of the recommendations made by this group was to translate the Standard to American English. The Standard as published for the North American market includes in the appendix the list of allergens required by law to be labelled in North America rather than the requirements of EU law. This attracted some comment from the UK Technical Advisory Committee who interpreted the inclusion of the North American allergen list in the Standard, as a change to the standard. However given the potential size of the food market in the US, BRC considered this an appropriate step. This issue highlights the problem that manufacturers have across the world when producing foods for many different markets

4.5 Integrity of Audits

One of the potential problems associated with third party schemes is lack of consistency of audits which is dependent on the effectiveness of the Accreditation process across the world. The National Accreditation Bodies have a responsibility to ensure that certification bodies are consistently operating the schemes for which they are accredited. The BRC recognises that that is a major task, and as the Standard owner, that maintaining the integrity of the scheme needs more direct input, from ourselves to ensure the consistency of audits.

In order to enhance the integrity of the BRC Standard, the BRC have tightened the auditor qualifications and training requirements. A fundamental review of the BRC training provision is underway to ensure BRC training providers undergo more stringent assessment, in addition the content of our training programmes is being reviewed.

The BRC directory is a web-based system that will provide access for all users of BRC certification schemes with access to the sites that have been approved. When a site has been certificated, the audit report can be made available to potential customers. A crucial element of the new directory is an auditor registration programme. All certification bodies now have to register their auditors with the BRC. There will be an automatic electronic check between the auditor that has produced the audit report, their qualifications, and the scope of products within those audits.

A newly appointed BRC compliance manager is responsible for closer liaison with the certification bodies, and surveillance monitoring of audit reports. The directory provides a communication process for the participants in the BRC Standard; the 14,000 certificated sites; 90 certification bodies; and 90 approved trainers. Monthly bulletins containing information to improve the integrity of the scheme are now being produced for all these involved parties. Any organisation must have a capture system for customer complaints, and the BRC has developed a feedback and complaints investigation process, so that if anyone has any concern about a BRC audit that they have had themselves, or that they have seen at a supplier that they have visited, whether that is an ingredient supplier or a supplier to a retailer, the BRC can be informed and investigate accordingly.

The BRC will also be working with stakeholders to identify what more needs to be done in terms of auditor training. We have placed a number of training obligations on auditors; such as Lead Assessor training, HACCP and 'How to Implement the BRC Global Standard'. We are considering whether there should be formal compulsory training on allergen management for BRC auditors.

4.6 Governance of the BRC Schemes Internationally

As the BRC schemes extend internationally we are also expanding our Governance structures accordingly. International input has been widened on the Governance and Strategy Committee; there is now representation from the United States and Australia. There are International Technical Advisory Committees who provide much more detailed information on the technical issues that are affecting their own countries, which are in place in Australia, and the United States. There are also international Certification Body Co-operation Groups where certification bodies within countries come together to discuss issues of relevance regarding compliance, interpretation and implementation of the Standard. These co-operation groups operate in the UK, North America, Australia, Spain, Germany and Italy. The BRC are working with the International Accreditation Forum to develop requirements for the Accreditation Bodies to improve the robustness of the accreditation process.

4.7 Provision of Information

The recently launched BRC Global Standards website may in future function as a focal point for technical information relating to particular topics. This could include an allergens section that details the legislation in different countries. We also plan to produce a Guideline on Good Allergen Management to assist the management of allergen containing materials more effectively

In the future the BRC will monitor international agencies as legislation and understanding on this issue converges, and will be looking to develop a common system for risk assessment and allergen management through standards and guidelines of appropriate detail.

4.8 Conclusion

We have heard much today about different approaches to assuring that sites manage allergens effectively. We believe that the BRC provides a firm basis for good allergen management. We are constantly looking to improve the information we supply to certificated sites and the integrity of audits. We are willing to work with any party or organisation to move to a common approach – to avoid duplication and cost and provide greater protection for the consumer.

5. ALLERGENS: BUILDING THE FOUNDATIONS FOR A ROBUST PROGRAMME

Deryck Tremble
AIB International

5.1 Introduction

This chapter will cover best practices and pre-requisite programmes, and also for more of a global perspective, some information will be provided from other parts of the world such as the United States. This chapter will also talk about the control of allergens, and the practical point of view.

It is very important to know how allergens are managed in other countries, particularly if a company is exporting, and language differences are also important to understand, in order that there is clarity in the practices and management of allergens required between one country and another. Language is important to recognise as a possible area for confusion when communicating technical issues to colleagues and clients in other countries; event though Americans speak English, there are distinct differences in terminology used between the two countries, and a certain amount of "translation" is required for messages to be clearly understood. An example of this is the use of the term cross-contact, which is the new buzzword for cross-contamination used more outside of the UK.

In the food industry, allergen control procedures that are in place and being applied in food factories are normally very good. In general in Europe, the documentation accompanying allergen control programmes is very good, but carrying out an inspection in the food plant reveals a very different picture. This is similar to the theory and practice of HACCP plans; what is written in the HACCP plan is not necessarily what is actually being done at the factory level.

It is important to understand that each allergen should be treated individually. More and more factories now will have an allergen warehouse, an allergen store, a sensitive ingredient area, but sometimes the cross-contamination issues in these areas are a cause for serious concern; sometimes, staff forget what they should be doing to keep those allergens away from each other.

Components of an allergen management programme are listed in Figure 5.1.

Programme Components
Allergen Identification
Receiving
Storage
Formula Control
Personnel Practices
Production Controls
Changeover Cleaning
Labelling
Engineering
Supplier Control
Research & Development
Quality Control
Purchasing
Education / Training
AIB

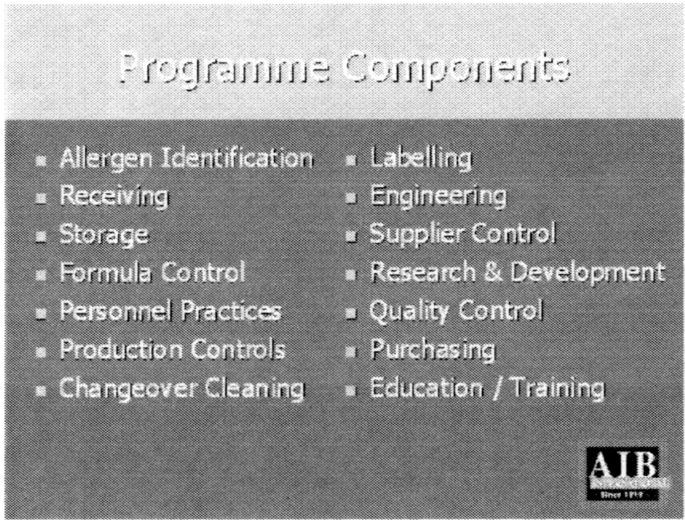

Fig. 5.1. Components of an Allergen Control Programme

5.2 Allergen Identification

Allergen identification is just one of the list of components of an allergen plan. Ingredients statements should be provided for all materials, and allergens should also be identified on the specification sheets for the products actually being produced on site. Specification sheets containing allergens should be clearly marked and readily identifiable (printed on specific coloured paper), and should include all by-products such as whey or casein derived from milk.

These are some of the best practices that should be in place as companies are focussing to ensure that people who are actually inside the facility are well aware of any allergens being used. When factory floor operatives are trained in allergen management, very, very few people don't understand the issues; quite often in a group of about 20 people, one will be able to talk about their little boy or their grandson that suffers because of peanut allergy for example.

5.3 Receiving Goods

When goods and ingredients are received, deliveries should be well controlled, with proper segregation of allergenic and non-allergenic materials on the same truck. Wash tickets or load histories should be obtained for bulk deliveries to exclude non-compatible materials. Identification of these allergen-control materials at receipt is essential. Colour coding the allergenic products with tags or other distinguishable means can be used very well, and this system is used in the

UK and the rest of Europe in particular. The ingredient declaration should always be reviewed, and companies should be aware of any changes made by their supplier.

5.4 Allergen Storage

All efforts are needed to avoid cross-contamination while in storage. Allergens should be stored with "like over like". All allergen-containing facilities should be at floor level if possible. That is not always possible, and sometimes the "sensitive ingredient area", as is the name for the area used to store allergenic ingredients, is too small to deal with all the perceived allergens, or sensitive ingredient materials that companies are currently using. One common trend is for very good ingredients control when the business is operating as normal, but as soon as anything out of the normal operating schedule occurs, such as a promotion, or special edition of a product, whereby the formulation changes, normal controls may not be adhered to closely enough. Such a promotion may be led by the marketing department, who suggest, for example, adding cheese and ham to a bread product, to increase sales. The initial issues will be with food quality and food safety, but allergen control is also a part of the equation, and should not be overlooked.

Allergen stores are sometimes not properly managed, and when this happens, spillages, and open boxes, are obviously sources of cross-contamination of ingredients. Control is much better when allergens are segregated in different areas. As an example, sesame seeds are very easily spread in a factory, and despite having a thorough clean down, it's highly likely that a subsequent inspection will locate some sesame seeds in the production plant.

5.5 Rework

More and more companies are taking the decision not to use any rework in their products, or they develop very complex equations, to calculate how rework can be incorporated to follow full traceability. Rework should only be used "like into like". All rework containers should be clearly labelled, and rework containing allergens should only be allowed on the factory floor during the current run of that product.

5.6 Personnel Practices

Personnel practices are essential to control the transfer of allergens, and hand washing with soap and water is essential to limit cross-contamination. Staff should wear the proper uniform, the movement around the factory of people working with allergens should be strictly controlled, and the potential of contamination from ingredients used in the canteen should be considered. In some instances, there is better control in the canteen than in the factory; for example many companies don't allow chocolate bars in the canteen that contain peanuts, but in the facility there is lots and lots of potential for cross-contact.

5.7 Production Controls

More and more companies are using dedicated lines for some allergen-containing products, even dedicated factories if the product is made at a multisite operation. Dedicated containers, scoops, and other utensils, that are colour-coded for easy identification are all advisable. The evidence of this level of thought into allergen control is easy to see when auditing a supplier. Flow patterns for all the allergen-containing products are important; a map for the location of all the allergens should be developed, for example, in the raw material warehouse, and more and more companies are developing an allergen matrix to help determine the order of their production runs. This very tight control is getting more difficult as more and more companies run their factories 24 hours a day. There isn't the 2-day weekend break that there used to be in the past, with consolidation of plant; more and more companies are running 24/7 and so allergen control and cleaning control have to go hand in hand.

There are various measures that can be put in place in terms of having a good schedule and ensuring the minimum amount of change-overs of production runs, and formula control is important. All the formulas containing allergens must be identified, and batch sheets or formula cards should be colour-coded for the allergens they contain. Rework must be identified to ensure like into like, and all other rework must be removed from the production floor. Lots of times, companies will make their allergen-containing products at the end of the day, and allow for thorough clean out times. Where issues can arise with the effectiveness of cleaning programmes is when companies are busy during times that a promotion is running, and the cleaning time goes down from half an hour to perhaps five minutes, or maybe 2 hours normally, down to half an hour, and this reduction in time for this important task is not sufficient for it to be done properly. It is when systems that are normally used are not followed that problems can occur with cross-contamination, which could lead to a product recall, or more importantly, could be fatal for someone.

5.8 Cleaning

Cleaning is crucial to the elimination of allergens from production equipment, and therefore preventing cross-contamination. Cleaning must take place between all allergen and non-allergen production, and between formulas using different allergens. Cleaning should be effective enough to remove all product residues, and to ensure that this is the case, different allergens or different products may require specific cleaning procedures. The type of cleaning method used should be assessed for its suitability; for example, air hose cleaning is not acceptable for allergen cleaning, because compressed air makes allergen material airborne, resulting in additional cross-contamination potential. It should be remembered that visual inspections to assess the effectiveness of cleaning processes can be limiting, and testing for residual allergenic proteins should be carried out to validate the procedure. The cleaning programme should take into account splash zones, indirect product contact surfaces, and utensils. When production switches from an allergenic to a non-allergenic ingredient, cloth transfers or absorbent material in contact with allergenic material must be changed and laundered. Finally, check sheets to verify cleaning equipment should be filled in upon completion of each cleaning cycle.

Making sure that the equipment used to do the cleaning is itself clean is important; brushes that are used for cleaning pans can also accumulate allergenic material. Using a torch to inspect equipment post-cleaning will help to identify the areas that have been overlooked, and can be highlighted to the cleaning team in order to improve performance. There are lots of small spaces between joints etc. in production equipment that can harbour a build-up of allergens.

5.9 Validation

The Food Allergy Research and Resource Program (FARRP) at the University of Nebraska conducts a lot of research into allergens and allergen testing, and some of their test kits are listed in Figure 5.2. Testing should be conducted to assess the effectiveness of cleaning programmes in removing allergens between production runs.

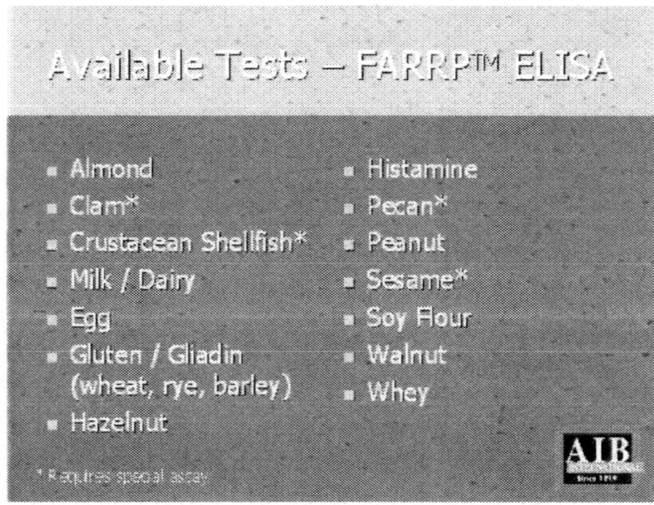

Fig. 5.2. Allergen test kits from FARRP

5.10 Allergen Labelling

In different parts of the world, there are different interpretations and focus on different types of allergens and perceived allergens. It is important that if a company is exporting to a country, the allergen labelling requirements of that country are understood. It is well known that 64% of product recalls are directly related to improper information on the labels, and a lot of that time the error can be traced back to the facility, and the change over in production. It is important that there is an ingredient review at the time of receipt of packaging materials, there should be verification of the label or packaging when it is introduced to the packaging line, there should be control of splicing mixed materials, and obsolete labels and packaging should be destroyed.

Statements that are used on labelling can be seen below, but are not an excuse for poor allergen management:

- "May Contain.........."
- "Manufactured on Equipment Used..........."
- "Manufactured in a Plant Where.........."
- "Product Contains...................."
- "....................Containing Product"

5.11 Engineering

Engineering strategies are needed to limit contamination from allergens via air movement, from line flow, at allergen addition points and in overall equipment design. If the design of processing equipment took into account how easy it is to clean, and minimized areas that product could build up, the risk of allergen cross-contamination could be significantly reduced.

5.12 Supplier Control

Regular contact with ingredients suppliers is very important. The suppliers control programme should include the same elements as the companies that they supply to. Requiring suppliers to complete a questionnaire to establish their allergen control procedures will help the receiving company manage the allergens in the final product. Examples of the questions asked are in Figure 5.3.

Specifications for the loading and transport of materials from a supplier should be provided to the supplier, because the product may be well controlled up to the point that it leaves the supplier, but what happens in that time in between, whether it is being stored in an off-site warehouse prior to being brought to the company purchasing it is important; it may be put into racks where there are other allergens that may not be well controlled.

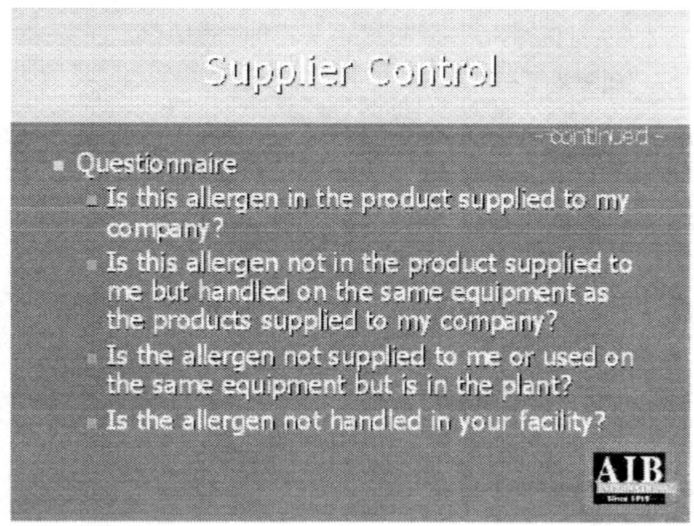

Fig. 5.3. Questions to ask of a Supplier

5.13 Research and Development

The team in research and development also have a role to play with respect to allergens. They can assist greatly by being keenly aware of those allergens already used on site, and formulating new products without adding new allergens. In one example, when conducting a factory audit, the production manager was very insistent that nuts were not used in the facility, yet there was a container found on the floor that contained nut paste, and was attributed to an R&D project. The equipment that the R&D team run tests on in the plant may not routinely come into contact with a particular allergen that may have been present in the test run, and therefore R&D should notify plant personnel ahead of time to ensure proper control before production runs start.

Quality Control personnel should also ensure that when raw materials are sampled in the warehouse, they are sealed correctly to ensure that spillage doesn't occur. Substitute ingredients should also be monitored closely to ensure that a new allergen is not introduced into a product.

Education and training are very, very important. People understand about food safety and about allergens, but their awareness needs to be raised. A lot of the time the food industry talks about tonnage, pallets, and number of packs. It is easy to lose sight of the fact that a small pack is going to be eaten by a five year old.

A company should establish control, assess its plant risks, have a good control programme in place, and continue to develop that. The company should raise allergen awareness on a regular basis, conduct allergen audits, evaluate its programme on a regular basis, in the same way that a HACCP programme would be reviewed, and make sure improvement changes are implemented and that they are effective.

6. STANDARDS, ESPECIALLY ALLERGEN CONTROL, AUDITS, INTERNAL INSPECTIONS AND THIRD PARTY

John Figgins,
Chemistry Manager
Sainsbury's Supermarkets Ltd

6.1 Introduction

Picture a scene: it's Saturday morning, a bank holiday weekend, and unusually this is a Saturday when you can have a leisurely breakfast, and as you pick up your second cup of tea and open your newspaper that's been conveniently delivered, you notice the headline on the front page is about another food scare. As you read the headline you wonder vaguely who has had their Saturday spoilt by this latest scare. Idly you turn to page 5 to see the full story, and start reading the details. And perhaps your pulse starts to quicken a little, maybe there is even an amount of perspiration on your brow as you realise that actually the products you produce could possibly be implicated. None of us would like to be in that scenario. Not on a Saturday morning, not at any time.

Good allergen management is a key aspect of product management; something that all food companies must aim for; safe products for the end consumer.

Sainsburys' goal is to 'exceed customers' expectations for healthy, safe, fresh & tasty food'. The wording used by other companies might be slightly different, but the motivation will be the same; food companies need to make foods that are safe, that have got the correct allergen controls in place.

6.2 Standards

Product safety can be viewed as a pyramid structure, with each layer of controls supporting all the others, so that overall the end product is safe. The diagram in Figure 6.1 clearly shows that standards and policies form the foundation on which other safety mechanisms can be built.

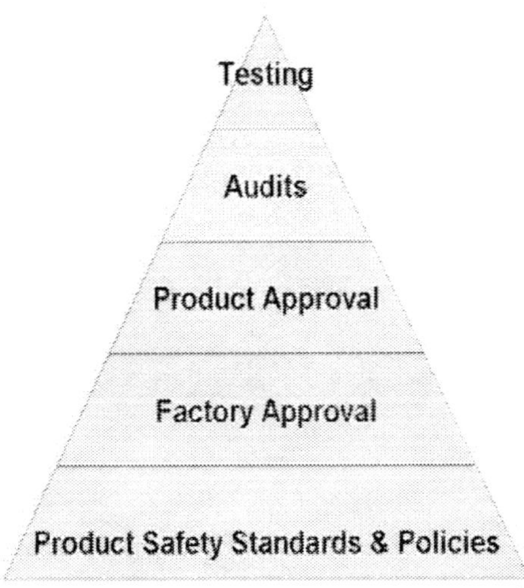

Fig. 6.1. Product Safety Pyramid

A relevant analogy from Sunday School is the story of a wise man who built his house on a stable rock, the idea being that when things went wrong the stable foundation was strong enough to support the house. In the same way, the wise factory manager will build their product safety and therefore their allergen controls on a stable foundation of good policies. Of course those policies need to have the right depth, the right detail, and the right robustness, and it is important to note that while a policy can be fantastic, if it is in the office gathering dust until the next audit then it is not being effective. Standards and food safety policies must be living, working documents implemented in everything that's actually happening in the factory; everything from raw material sourcing, to the product leaving the store. If food safety policies are not influencing all the stages, then they are just dry documents.

The BRC Global Standard Issue 5 makes allergen control a fundamental requirement, and defines fundamental as "systems that are crucial to the establishment and operation of an effective food quality and safety operation". The BRC Standard lists eight areas which effectively cover the manufacturing process. These can be summarised as:

- The need to carry out risk assessments of raw materials
- Identification of all allergens on site
- Risk assessment of routes of cross-contamination and documented procedures to avoid contamination.
- Procedures to manage re-work

- Validation of production procedures to substantiate allergen claims
- Risk assessment and validation of cleaning procedures
- Staff training
- Management of non-conformities

Every company in the food industry must have a formal policy on allergen control. This policy should outline the company's position on allergens, its aims; what it is trying to achieve with its products. For manufacturers it also needs to detail the procedures and controls required for every step of production.

6.3 HACCP

In developing a policy to manage allergens, a HACCP system should be applied. HACCP plans are an established tool, known to work for other aspects of food safety. Hazard analysis using a HACCP-based system must therefore be in place to determine the necessary activities to manage allergens, track their location and identify and control any cross-contamination. It is obvious that every single part of the process must be covered in the allergen HACCP plan, it is somewhat inevitable that any element not included in the plan, whether intentionally or accidentally, will be the one that causes problems with allergens at a later date.

Pre-requisite programmes must also be considered. In the area of allergen management, the pre-requisite programme is often effectively used as a critical control. For example, if cleaning is relied upon for allergen control, then, even if it is in the pre-requisite programme, it has got to be thorough, it has got to be effective, it has got to be documented and it has got to be validated.

Figure 6.2 shows examples of the areas an allergen HACCP plan must cover:

- Consider the entire process
  - Raw material receipt & storage
  - Scheduling
  - Weighing up
  - Production
  - Cleaning
  - Packing Line
  - Storage
- Validation & documentation
- Pre-requisite programme

Fig. 6.2. Example Requirements for a Manufacturer's Allergen HACCP

The issue of potential allergen cross contamination requires special consideration, focus and attention, and the resultant policies will again need to be documented and validated.

6.4 Allergen Free Products

Sainsbury's have a range of Freefrom products which make allergen free claims. Some parts of the industry have expressed concerns with the concept of allergen free claims; however they remain popular with allergic customers, especially wheat, gluten and dairy free ranges. Allergen free products will attract allergic customers, the most susceptible and vulnerable customers, with the assurance that the products are definitely safe for them, and it is therefore critical to have an additional set of controls in place, once the allergen free claim is made. These added controls will need to manage exactly where the specified allergens are, that they are properly segregated, that further staff training has taken place, additional management of the production line and minimisation of staff movement. This is best done by producing allergen free foods in dedicated factories.

There will be extra testing validation requirements, to justify the use of the allergen free claim on the food with confidence that the product is and remains safe for its target audience.

6.5 Audits

Audits are a vital part of the allergen control process, both internal audits and those from an external body, be they second or third party, because they will form part of the validation of a company's processes. The whole system needs to be audited at regular points. An audit conducted by an external auditor will try to cover as much of the process as possible in the allotted time. For an internal inspection it may be a valid and better use of resource to inspect certain parts of the process at different times, and schedule them accordingly.

There are a range of elements that must be included in audits, from raw material sourcing, through to production. It is important not to overlook engineering, and new product development (NPD). These are 2 key departments that can be implicated in problems with allergens. For example, it is not unknown for factory Technical Managers to be surprised by the ingredients the NPD team have started to use. If the factory is nut free does the NPD department really understand what this means for them? Therefore, involving and communicating with the NPD team is vital to ensure that allergen management policies are followed across the site.

When audits are conducted, there are 2 questions that should be considered:

1. Are the Standards applied in practice, rather than being a document sitting unused in an office?

2. Does the Standard being applied by the business actually deliver the required outcome in terms of allergen control?

Figure 6.3 shows examples of the areas that must be verified as part of an allergen audit:

- Raw Material Sourcing, Controls & Storage
- Customer complaints and other incidents of non-conforming product, including investigation & formal review of such products and instigation of appropriate corrective action
- Production Processes & Controls
- Personnel (including Movement, Equipment Usage & Training)
- Work in Progress (including Identification, Management & Re-work)
- Non-conformance management (including Spillage, Incident Reporting and Investigations)
- Engineering (including Materials, Cross-Contamination, Equipment Maintenance and Movement)

Fig. 6.3. Example Aspects of Allergen Auditing and Verification

6.6 Conclusions

Despite having Standards in place and continuing to apply them, as an industry numerous brands have suffered allergen-related product withdrawals and recalls resulting from allergens being in the wrong product. For example, on one occasion Sainsbury's had to initiate a product recall for two types of chilled cheesecake. Whilst the information on the packaging was correct, on the implicated date of production the manufacturer used the wrong recipe card and therefore the wrong ingredients. This resulted in the presence of undeclared egg in the product.

This case, and the many similar ones that are reported, suggest that even the simple controls need further work, further depth and further robustness to deliver standards that are rigorously and continuously delivered in the factory.

7. SUPPLY AND FACTORY CONTROL

Terry Wilde, Product Integrity Manager
Tesco Foods

This presentation will cover: ingredient supply; storage; processing; and right product / wrong packet.

7.1 Ingredient Supply

Several years ago, while working as a Technical Manager for a UK retailer I was called by a hospital who had admitted a young child following reaction to a food purchased at one of our stores. The hospital asked me if our product contained peanuts. The product didn't contain peanuts; however other nuts were present in the recipe. Clearly we were concerned and an investigation was undertaken. As part of the investigation we went to visit the raw material supplier of the nuts to better understand their facility. The visit identified that the nut supplier also handled peanuts, and the manufacturer of our product was not aware of this fact. Although this event took place a number of years ago, issues such as this (where an allergen appears in a product because of an error further back in the supplier chain), are still occurring.

Manufacturers and retailers need to know what goes into their products. Accurate, detailed specifications are a necessity. Factory audits continue to establish that some companies do not have detailed specifications for all raw materials. Tesco, as a responsible retailer, expects a manufacturer of their brand to have a detailed specification for every product that they make.

It is a requirement that manufacturers understand how their suppliers are operating; what activities they undertake, and whether they are handling certain allergenic ingredients. The Tesco view is that physical audits are the best way to determine these facts; however, taking a practical approach, it is understood that it is very difficult for each manufacturer to audit every single raw material supplier, and therefore, a risk based approach is required.

Clearly not all manufacturers audit their suppliers and a significant number of them use agents, traders and distributors. The relationship that an agent, trader or distributor has with a product is most likely geared toward selling it, rather than producing it. It would be justifiable therefore to question how much detailed knowledge these intermediaries have about the products they are supplying and the factories that these originate from, e.g. have they been to the specific factory manufacturing the prodcut and have they verified that the product specification is accurate? If not, how much reliance can be placed upon the information provided?

A recent survey conducted by a data management company (collating data from supplier questionnaires and raw material specifications) indicated that 28% of the raw material suppliers participating in this data management program could not provide an allergen management policy when challenged. Approximately 8% of the specifications submitted were rejected due to insufficient allergen data. Agents, traders and distributors are supplying a lot of this information and it would appear that a number of the individuals involved do not fully understand their products or the requirements on handling allergens. This data may not be a true reflection of the UK food industry as a whole, but certainly provides an indication that there may be a significant gap between the expectations regarding allergen management and the reality of the situation.

Any manufacturer producing a Tesco brand product must know what goes into that product. This includes having detailed knowledge of suppliers for all the raw materials that the product contains. Where agents, traders or distributors are used by these manufacturers to supply raw materials, then the manufacturer is expected to have this information either by auditing the agent (to be confident that the agent's own systems are robust) or by auditing the supplying facility. It is essential that the information provided is accurate and a true reflecction of the supplying site.

7.2 Storage

A lot of the guidance about correct the storage of allergenic materials is mainly common sense. It is often overlooked but the physical form of the raw material is important, as it can obviously present different hazards and therefore needs to be handled appropriately. Milk as an allergen can be present in many forms e.g. it is more likely that milk powder will be spilled when used, than milk in the form of a block of cheese. This fact must be taken into account when conducting risk assessments relating to the allergens handled on a manufacturing site.

As mentioned, the storage of allergens in reality is relatively simple. Allergens must be clearly labelled, should not be stored in racking above other products, and cleaning to remove allergens should be efficient and effective. Detailed procedures must be in place to aid compliance. Staff training is crucial, to ensure this occurs, and that there is an understanding of the necessity of the procedure and the consequences of non-compliance. In reality there is little point in having detailed procedures in place, if people are not sufficiently trained to adhere to them.

Tesco have detailed requirements, but in simple terms: manufacturers must consider how they identify allergen;, how they decant allergens from a secure storage area; how they handle part-used bags / boxes containing allergens; and how they transfer allergens to manufacturing areas. Manufacturers should also consider whether the training given is really effective.

7.3 Processing

It is Tesco's perception that there is a lack of advice on 'best practice' for managing allergens. The majority of training providers ensure that delegates are provided with data on the number of people who suffer from allergies; detailing incidents involving individuals who regrettably have died from an allergic reaction and the frequent reporting of such incidents in the media. Clearly the emphasis is placed on the food industry to manage the allergen issue effectively or face the damaging consequences of failure. There however, appears to be a lack of information available to the food industry on how best to deal effectively with the allergen issue.

Manufacturing sites still face significant issues when dealing with large numbers of allergens or having facilities and products not suited to frequent 'wet cleaning'.

Sites need an effective allergen management programme that is understood and supported by all the senior management at a manufacturing facility. Tesco expects as a minimum that manufacturers understand what allergens are present on their site, what products those allergens go into, and which products do not contain allergens. Surprisingly, supplier auditing has established that on occasions these simple requirements are not always met.

It should be clear which production lines the allergen-containing products are made on, and the form of the allergen should be understood, for example, is it milk powder, or is it a block of cheese. These are all important in establising effective allergen management. Tesco expects that manufacturers will do their utmost to prevent allergen cross-contamination, and doesn't believe that 'may contain' labelling justifies poor allergen controls. It is clear that 'may contain' labelling is seen to be an insurance policy against poor factory management

Tesco has debated internally whether a hierarchy of allergens would be beneficial; is one allergen more of a problem than another allergen? There is no clear answer to that question yet. Accepted data on thresholds is not currently available and sufferers of milk allergy would not agree that crustaceans are more of an issue. What is clear however is that where sites use a large number of different allergens, it is not practical to have a large number of different colour coding systems in place to manage them effectively. It can be justifiably argued that the more complex the system to control the allergens, the greater the potential for misunderstanding by factory operatives, along with the associated consequences. However, all food manufacturing sites should have a policy in place to manage allergens.

At the beginning of this section it was indicated that there is a lack of information on how best to deal effectively with allergens in the manufacturing environment. This continues to pose the biggest challenge to the food industry.

As a company Tesco is not going to dictate what is categorically the right approach, but we are listening to our suppliers, and working with them across a range of industry sectors. We would like to issue practical guidance on allergen management that can be effectively implemented. We having been working with both large and small companies on this project and have encountered numerous issues. Where allergens are identified at very low levels it is difficult to determine if this has the potential to cause an allergic reaction. Clearly having reaction thresholds would be helpful, because the food industry could at least tackle the problem of allergen management in order of significance to the consumer. At present the industry is currently trying to prevent all possible cross contamination and in reality this is not proving to be an effective approach.

To summarise, we recognise that effective allergen management is problematic, especially for industries that have historically not wet cleaned on a daily basis. All food manufacturing sites must however, have a comprehensive allergen management programme in operation, and this will need to be challenged regularly to determine that it is effective.

7.4 Right Product Wrong Packet

Putting the right product in the wrong packet has been an issue for years. The implications are now more serious with respect to allergens, but it used to be an issue about the right meat pie in the wrong vegetarian packaging. Clearly there has been a noticeable increase in product recalls classified as 'allergen related' but in reality these are not all fundamentally about allergen control. Previously they may still have occurred, but would not have been classified as an allergen issue at the time. Clearly allergens relate to food safety, so have to be taken extremely seriously.

Food manufacturers need to assess their factories and the products they produce to determine the potential for future problems. For example sites may wish to consider the following when producing similar looking products containing different allergens:

- Can the product be made distinctive? - frozen pies often look similar and a different lid pattern may help distinguish them
- Can products be stored in different coloured containers (labelled) if intermediate / work in process stages are used?
- Is there potential for similar-looking packaging to be mixed up in storage areas or on packing equipment? Can product cartons / sleeves be delivered / stored in different-coloured liners?
- The language and reading ability of production operatives (particularly where a number of different nationalities are employed) can be a problem.
- If agency workers are utilised, have they had sufficient training and should certain tasks such as obtaining packaging or materials be restricted?

Clearly the list of possible problems is extensive but companies need to review which particular issues are applicable to their manufacturing sites and determine whether they have addressed them effectively.

8. I WANT IT ALL AND I WANT IT NOW! ALLERGY INFORMATION FOR CUSTOMERS

Moira Howie, Company Nutritionist
Waitrose Ltd

8.1 Introduction

In an ideal world I would like to report that Waitrose have never been involved in a product recall, however; the day before the Leatherhead Allergy Conference in May 2009, Waitrose was involved in a product recall, which involved an oriental supper for two. It was a classic case of the right product in the wrong packaging, which of course, is an increasingly common cause for product recalls. The allergens present in the meal are milk, peanuts, fish and shellfish. Any product recall involves communicating with consumers, and Waitrose has processes in place to deal with such a recall.

The title of this chapter "I want it all and I want it now" really does sum up today's consumers and their expectations with respect to food information. As a retailer, Waitrose expects a detailed level of information about products from its suppliers, particularly when a product recall occurs. Information needs to be made available as quickly as possible so that in turn, consumers can be supplied with the best information. Consumers' expectations have risen enormously; they expect that all food should be safe to eat, and this extends to allergy status, with all information about allergens in foods being clear and concise. The ideal of course is to offer the allergic consumer exactly the same level of choice that a non-allergic consumer would want to see in a supermarket, unfortunately; that has become increasingly difficult as the supply base begins to consolidate, and there are less options available to retailers.

Waitrose strive to make sure that any information on the label is clear and wherever possible does not contain ambiguous statements. If there is an error, we need to be able to explain very quickly and very clearly to the customer what that issue might be so that they can either return the product, make an informed choice, or indeed throw the product away if that is what they choose to do.

8.2 Entertaining at Home

Eating outside the home for allergy sufferers is still something of a gamble, when it comes to communicating special dietary needs to restaurant staff, and being certain that the final food served is suitable to eat. Waitrose has been able to tap into the need for customers who want to entertain at home in the same way that you would do if you went out to a restaurant.

Waitrose were the first retailer to put full allergy information in the food section of its Food and Home brochure, which is available in all stores, and is a service available for people who want to entertain at home.

Naturally when ordering products to feed several people, it is important to know all of the allergens present because you may well be entertaining a range of guests with differing dietary requirements. Information on all of the key allergens is provided in the brochure, and of course the more allergens that are added to products, the more information the brochure contains which in turn makes it increasingly difficult to manage. At Waitrose we want to provide reassurance to the customer and to our partners, the people that serve in store, that the information they give to customers is correct. We would be letting our customers down if they opened their products at a picnic or party and realised that there is nothing for the milk and egg allergic consumer to eat, or that a product has nuts or gluten present and one of the guests is allergic to those ingredients.

This type of brochure goes to print several weeks before it appears in stores, so all of the technical information from all of the specifications of the products in the brochure must thoroughly checked for their allergy status long before the consumer purchases any of the products. This can be as long as 10, sometimes 12 weeks before this information goes in to print. The brochure is produced 3 times a year, and at Christmas there is added impetus to deliver the brochure to stores well in advance of the festive occasion. Waitrose's goal is to try to communicate very clearly with customers and to make sure the information is up to date, and not out of date once it goes into store. Occasionally this does happen, and that creates an additional set of problems, because there are many tens of thousands of brochures printed and distributed to customers.

8.3 Free from Lists

There has been a lot of discussion about 'may contain traces of nuts', and nuts are by far the most controversial allergen for all consumers. That is because it has been very well documented that fatalities do occur; of course fatalities are not just related to consumption of nuts, fatalities have been related to eggs and shellfish, but allergy incidents related to nuts have certainly received the most coverage.

Gluten is the most popular free-from list that is requested by our customers, showing that gluten is still a very important allergen. Clearly gluten consumption for coeliac sufferers causes great discomfort if they are exposed to gluten and don't know it, but in general the condition is an intolerance, and therefore it will not cause a fatal reaction. Waitrose's free-from lists are very popular, and as an organisation Waitrose is beginning to be concerned about offering free-from lists, because the very words in themselves place the company in an awkward position. The lists are intended to help allergic consumers in that they are a "positive" list of foods that consumers can buy based on the allergen status. Waitrose is supplying these lists with the best possible knowledge that these products are understood to be free from milk, egg, and gluten. Unfortunately there are no absolute guarantees, because of some of the issues in allergen management and what happens in the factory on any given day.

As this goes to print the discussions on exact wording centre around the avoidance of the words 'free from gluten' and are moving to 'suitable for those avoiding gluten'.

8.4 May Contain

The use of the term 'may contain traces of nuts' is used for a reason, and Waitrose do rely quite heavily on self-help groups like the Anaphylaxis Campaign to educate customers about why these statements should be taken seriously. Waitrose collaborate with the Anaphylaxis Campaign in the event of needing to communicate with those customers who should be informed if products have a change of allergy status. The Anaphylaxis Campaign put the information on their website, Waitrose put a statement on their website, and the FSA also put it on their website, creating a cascade of information that is put into place fairly quickly in order to help customers avoid any disastrous consequences of consuming a product that is no longer suitable for them.

8.5 Waitrose Product Recall Management

So what is the Waitrose approach when the situation of right product, wrong packaging arises? A 4-pronged approach is used.

1) Shelf-edge tickets in store display appropriate information, so that anybody buying that product is alerted straight away to the fact there has been a change in the allergy status of that product. The shelf-edge ticket mechanism is really important for informing customers. Figure 8.1 provides an example of wording used to alert customers . This was issued as a direct result of a change in factory status.

Important Notice for Nut & Sesame Allergy Sufferers
Due to supplier issues a number of ready prepared foods have moved production site. Please check the allergen panel on pack which will now state 'may contain traces of nuts and sesame'.

Fig. 8.1. Example of shelf ticket information

This sort of situation is disappointing, but these things have to happen in order to help Waitrose suppliers consolidate some production lines; however it does mean that the nut allergic customers have their choice of products further reduced.

2) The use of direct mail and pro-active letters to inform people who are specifically allergic, through self-help groups like the Anaphylaxis Campaign and Allergy UK who have very comprehensive databases, and are able to target those customers that need the information most.

3) The use of Waitrose website, which needs to display the change in allergy status on all products affected. Despite the fact that the products don't actually contain nuts, the nature of the allergy control is changing, which means that the technical specification then has to state 'may contain traces of nuts'. The other element of the business that is affected is the Food and Home brochure, so the implications of a few products changing production line have a knock-on effect in the shop, in the brochure, and when ordered online. What might appear to be a very simple change from a supplier point of view actually starts a cascade and chain of events for customer communication across a number of vehicles throughout the business.

4) The information on pack should change to reflect the new allergen status. In the current climate where the cost of packaging dictates that the Company don't write off packaging unnecessarily, the existing packaging would be used up. To facilitate this we add a sticker to the pack to alert customers. Naturally the packaging would be updated as soon as possible.

8.6 Sourcing

Waitrose have become increasingly global with sourcing suppliers. The BRC 5th version of their Standard is an invaluable tool for auditing suppliers, but these are not the only standards. Tesco and Sainsbury's both indicated that they have additional requirements of their suppliers, and Waitrose have these in place too. Suppliers dedicated to exclusive supply are much more difficult to find, and increasingly retailers are sharing the supply base, with large numbers of suppliers providing to all the main retailers.

The raw material suppliers are offering fewer guarantees for individual retailers, and the whole allergen management picture gets increasingly complicated with a faster moving culture of promotions, and greater pressure to produce multiple products on production lines that may previously only have happened during seasonal periods.

So there is consolidation of the supply base for many retailers and this includes Waitrose; these economies of scale put added pressures on the issues that need to be managed in the factory, such as allergens.

To finish I want to profile a case study of allergen management on dried mango, which happened at the end of 2008. This is a product that Waitrose sell all year round; it comes through a European supplier, and there are additional products packed on the line normally used for the mango, at Christmas, when there is significant uplift for dried fruit and nuts. The supplier had met the full audit requirements, BRC and our additional requirements.

A customer purchased a pack of dried mango, completely sealed and in transparent packaging. The contents included a hazelnut, a pistachio shell, and a cranberry, thankfully there was mango too! The customer alerted the Anaphylaxis Campaign and they in turn contacted us to investigate. The product was labelled with ‘may contain traces of nuts and sesame’. This is not something done routinely on every pack, but because it was a product that was being packed during the Christmas period it was felt that there was an additional risk of nut contamination occurring, and the defensive labelling was felt to be appropriate in this case. The result was a website alert issued via the Anaphylaxis Campaign. There was clearly a packaging contents error, but Waitrose, together with the Anaphylaxis Campaign wanted to alert people to the fact that these statements are not used indiscriminately despite what customers might think. They are only used when a very real risk exists, and that risk showed itself to be true at this point in time. The opportunity that the Anaphylaxis Campaign took was to remind all those with severe food allergies that these alerts should be taken seriously, especially with an increase in these statements. As a result sufferers start to ignore them, at their peril, and particularly in the younger members of the population, who perhaps are a little bit more glib, and think “I’ve eaten this with ‘may contains’ on many times” with no adverse reaction. Unfortunately, the next time could prove fatal. So people should not ignore these statements and start to consume products freely.

Like many manufacturers and retailers, Waitrose do not want to have to keep using ‘may contain’ statements on products, and Waitrose take it very seriously when the status of a product has to change.

The pack label is very limited in terms of space and companies can’t put all of the information that they might like to on there, so have to rely very heavily on other communication vehicles; the pack can not do it all. Lots of people aren't interested in reading the pack, they want a mobile phone message, they want it beamed to them through some ether, or other means, so there are a lot of different vehicles available in order to make sure that any allergy status is communicated, via as many avenues as possible.

So to summarise, indiscriminate use of 'may contain' statements is not desirable, but where they do appear, all customers should take them seriously, and the very important role that self-help groups like the Anaphylaxis Campaign play should not be underestimated; theirs is a very valued service, both to the food industry, and to the consumers that they serve. As a result of the value that Waitrose place on this service, all of Waitrose suppliers were asked to become corporate members of the Anaphylaxis Campaign so that they could also increase their own awareness and be linked into that very important vehicle for customer communication.

9. REGULATORY CONTROL

Jacqueline Ross, Chair,
Marks & Spencer Allergen Working Group

9.1 Introduction

Regulatory control underpins allergen management, and therefore how that is implemented within the supply base and finished products.

The list of major allergens is now well accepted and recognised by industry. A number of years ago, Marks and Spencer (M&S) Allergen Working Group, as part of an on-going horizon scanning exercise, (monitoring future trends and issues) identified lupin flour, and more specifically the protein in lupin flour, as an emerging allergen of concern due to the cross reactions suffered by those with nut allergy. M&S didn't use lupin as an ingredient at that time, and took the decision to ban its use in M&S products going forward. Looking back, that was the right decision to make as subsequently lupin was added to the EU Allergen List. One of the functions of the M&S Allergen working group is to monitor what is happening in industry, and the technical literature, in order to set policy, and ensure that suppliers are given in advance adequate information about decisions relating to allergens.

9.2 Allergen and May Contain Labelling

M&S do not sell snails, so have combined molluscs and crustaceans together under the category of shellfish to try and provide clear information to customers on the back of the pack. Labelling on M&S products has changed quite considerably over the past few years, based on really listening to what customers want. M&S has a set of labelling guidelines that all M&S suppliers can review on a website, and that changes as legislation changes. M&S also provides information on pack over and above legal requirements.

Examples of changes in allergen labelling on M&S products; historically the alibi labelling that stated whether a product had been made in a factory that handled nuts, used to appear before the box stating what allergens the product contained. This has been changed so that the "contains" box appears before the alibi labelling, because M&S felt that the "contains" information is far more important. The "contains" box is now also very clearly highlighted as containing allergen information. Not all M&S customers understood that the "contains" box related to the allergen information.

As with all the other major retailers, M&S uses 'may contain' labelling in relation to dark chocolate due to the possibility that it may contain milk or soya if milk chocolate is also made on the same production line. The statement 'This factory also manufactures milk chocolate and as a result this product may contain Milk and Soya' is used as it gives much more information to the customer as it has been very clearly proven that there can be a detectable level of milk present in dark chocolate.

M&S policy is to seek to minimise the use of warning (alibi) labels. While warning labels are used on some products, these are considered on a product by product basis. In circumstances where an alibi statement is deemed to be necessary, M&S will make sure that the supplier has conducted a full risk assessment. M&S has a number of codes of practice that relate to allergen management, one of which is about risk management and use of allergen management within the factories. If a supplier wishes to use an alibi label, they have to have completed five stages of risk assessment. Suppliers need to have completed an in-depth risk assessment looking at the products they are using on site, they need to have identified areas where they can improve that process to try and eliminate any of the risk, and if after that improvement plan has been implemented there is still a risk, that is when M&S will take the decision to use the alibi label. This decision involves the site technologist and also the Allergen Working Group. At the moment, M&S feel that this is the correct approach, and until there are allergen thresholds to work to, or at least action levels, this is the best means of minimising risk to customers.

One of the key aspects of our regulatory control and labelling guidelines is to make sure that we have the most accurate information going to our customers. As part of the new product development process, an external body is commissioned to verify and check all of our specifications, which generate pack copy and therefore the final product packaging. That means that there are suppliers, M&S staff and also an external body looking and checking specifications against product labelling so that no mistakes occur on the information provided on the final product. This is a robust checking system which has been in place since the beginning of 2008, and to date has been working very well.

9.3 Allergen Management Across the Business

M&S has a number of different formats for selling food to customers. In many cases customers can also consume food on the premises, which makes allergens extremely difficult to control. Safety when eating out is a very difficult aspect of living with a life-threatening allergy. M&S try to give as much information as possible; information on allergens is provided by in-store bakery and also in cases where the product is sold loose. M&S delicatessen bars and cafes have undergone more risk assessments to look at whether there is the right cleaning plan in place, whether products can be segregated, and whether there are separate staff; all the aspects that would be expected within manufacturing sites are applied back to our catering areas within store. M&S constantly review these risk assessments and amend working practices as relevant in light of any further information available on allergen management. All the factories that supply products to the delicatessen bars, restaurants and cafes, must still undergo full proper risk assessments; they must minimise any cross-contamination. There is no justification that if a product bears an alibi statement that the manufacturer can take less care; it should still be produced to exactly the same standards as all other products.

9.4 Free From Lists

The M&S web site contains allergy information relating to food products sold within its stores, and M&S are seeing a huge increase in requests for free-from lists, not only for gluten, but also dairy and egg as well. Customers can request free-from lists, but M&S actually name them "products that do not contain" in terms of the named ingredient, and it is very important to state this to customers. This information is updated every month and it is a requirement of M&S suppliers to ensure that their online specifications, which also drive packaging generation, are also up to date, as the 'do not contain' lists are automatically generated.

9.5 Product Recalls

The M&S Allergen Working Group monitors product recall information from alerts via the Food Standards Agency and also the mainland European Food Safety Authority, as well as looking at what's happening relating to allergens both in Europe, and in the UK. In 2008, allergens contributed to approximately 40% of the UK product withdrawals and recalls where the cause of these recalls, in many cases, was the wrong product in the wrong packaging.

Making sure that the right product is in the right packaging is a key area to focus on, and whilst errors of this type are decreasing, there are challenges faced by suppliers to avoid this mistake happening; M&S has several coordinated ranges, for example there might be two different products, with different allergen declarations, but the products look very similar, so it is difficult to tell the difference between the two. M&S suppliers have been asked to look at in-line automatic label verification, and there needs to be an extremely good case not to utilise these inline label verification systems, as a means of avoiding putting the wrong packaging on a product. A number of manufacturers already have these in place; they may be vision scans, 2D bar codes, or standard bar codes, but all these methods are effective in preventing many of the potential issues.

In a product recall of an M&S product in June 2008, the manufacturer did not have inline label scanning, the product had the correct top label, but the wrong base label. The base label was black and white, and looked essentially no different to the other labels used on site, this is an example of why M&S are asking companies to invest in inline verification to prevent situations such as this.

Another part of M&S labelling guidelines is that whenever a supplier makes a change to a product, be it one that might affect the allergen status or for any other reason, an improved recipe flash is always put on the front of pack. Despite what the design studio insists on what the pack looks like, or the use of any other promotional stickers, this information has to take precedence; this is very important because a new recipe flash should act as a prompt to customers that something has changed about the product and they should be looking at the ingredients list to see whether that affects them.

9.6 Allergenic Ingredients

The Anaphylaxis Campaign are extremely good at communicating allergen information with both the food industry and their corporate members in the food industry. One such alert gave information on a young milk-allergic boy who had died following an allergic reaction to milk in a pineapple and coconut juice drink. The milk was listed in the ingredients list, but the neither the boy nor his mother expected milk to be used in such a product. This highlights that consumers don't always think about what might be in a product, and don't always look at the back of pack, expecting the front of the product to tell them everything about it. M&S have taken this into account when labelling a new range of smoothies launched within their health drinks range. The front of the pack highlights use of omega-3 fish oil, and the decision was taken to highlight this on the front of the product, because it is not necessarily something that the customer might expect to be in a banana, date and oat probiotic dairy smoothie. This was a weighted risk as we also took into account customer perception that they might think it tastes of fish, and so not try the product. The presence of fish oil is also highlighted on the back of pack in the contains box, but the front of pack icon highlights the approach that M&S takes, to try not to put any unlikely ingredients in products without informing the customer. M&S suppliers are asked whether they have any products that contain allergens that might not be expected to be found in that type of product, and suppliers must then assess whether that allergen really needs to be in there. A good example of where ingredients have been changed is breaded ham, which used to have milk proteins in the bread coating, but these have been removed because it was felt that consumers wouldn't expect milk protein to be present in this type of product.

So ongoing from a regulatory point of view, manufacturers and retailers have to continue to be aware of what is happening with respect to allergens, both from the consumers' point of view, and also in the wider industry and across the world.

Knowledge and understanding of allergens is increasing and rapidly changing, and so presents a continued challenge all the time. The next challenge for the food industry will be around gluten free and the regulations on less than 20 ppm, which is going to have a significant impact on what is declared on products. The only free from products that M&S sells are gluten-free, and that is because gluten can be measured, all products in the range contain less than 20 ppm gluten; M&S do not currently sell any other positively labelled 'free-from' products because of the uncertainty about whether the foods are indeed free from particular allergens, and the difficulty of tracking back through the supply chain to be able to do adequate allergen testing.

10. ALLERGEN CLEANING PROJECT

Simon Flanagan
Head of Speciality Analysis & Allergen Services
Reading Scientific Services Limited (RSSL)

This chapter will cover the results of a study that was run in collaboration with the Reading Scientific Services Laboratory (RSSL) and the Anaphylaxis Campaign, which monitored the effects of different cleaning methods and their ability to remove residual allergenic proteins. This work was very much targeted at the catering sector.

10.1 Background

In 2006 RSSL ran a collaborative project in conjunction with the Anaphylaxis Campaign to investigate the effectiveness of different cleaning interventions and their effectiveness in removing allergens. It was decided that the study should focus on the catering sector given that the highest number of severe allergic reactions were experienced by sensitised consumers whilst eating away from home (Source Anaphylaxis Campaign). At the time it was largely unknown whether these reactions were due to negligence on behalf of the vendor, or whether there was an issue in terms of cross-contamination with shared utensils used in the catering kitchen. When designing this study it was also clear that there was a lack of robust published research in this area with the exception of a single study published in 2004 which assessed the removal of peanut proteins from school canteen surfaces (1).

In an attempt to try and address this knowledge gap RSSL designed a study to understand the efficacy of different wet cleaning regimes employed within the catering sector by mimicking residual allergen contamination on a range of different food contact surfaces. Although this study was very much aimed at the catering sector, there are some parallels which can be drawn with the wider food industry.

10.2 Objectives and Methods

This study had four main objectives:

1. To monitor the performance of different commercial Enzyme-Linked Immunsorbent Assays (ELISA) to detect residual allergenic proteins. The study compared three different peanut ELISA kits, two different hazelnut ELISA kits, and three different milk ELISA kits kindly supplied by Neogen, Biopharm Rhone, and Tepnel Biosystems.
2. To measure the tenacity of three different allergens. Hazelnut and peanut were chosen for the study because they are relatively prevalent allergies and their associated allergenic proteins are capable of eliciting reactions at extremely low levels. Milk was also chosen because it is a common allergy in the UK, and the associated allergenic proteins are biochemically very different to either the peanut or hazelnut proteins.
3. To monitor the effectiveness of cleaning methods, chemicals and materials in removing allergenic residues from artificially contaminated surfaces i.e. comparing the efficiency of allergen removal of bowl washing with a commercial detergent vs the performance of an automated wash in a commercial dishwasher.
4. To monitor the ease of cleaning of different physical contact surfaces, i.e. stainless steel, wood, polythene, etc. All of the surfaces and utensils chosen for this study were previously 'pre-used' in order to present the 'worst-case' scenario.

The allergenic simulants chosen for the study were National Institute of Standards and Technology (NIST)-Certified peanut butter; a commercial chocolate hazlenut spread and milk custard, prepared in the laboratory using certified milk powder. When assessing the data from all of the studies the results were normalised to account for the very different protein levels between the three simulants.

Pre-weighed amounts of each of the allergen simulants were placed on to glass fibre spreaders. A stencil was used for the application of simulant onto work surfaces and the chopping boards to ensure standard application over a fixed surface area. Following application of the simulants, work surfaces were left for approximately one hour to dry before proceeding to cleaning. For the cooking utensils (baking trays, pots and pans), the allergens were applied, and then the utensils were subjected to a heat treatment. Post heat treatment utensils were allowed to cool, and then cleaned using pre-defined methods. All of the utensils, chopping boards, pots and pans used for the study were all pre-used to mimic the 'worst case' scenario in a working environment. Once the work surfaces and utensils had been through individual standardised cleaning procedures, surface swabs were taken from each of the cleaned surfaces and tested for the respective allergen by ELISA. A number of the surface swab samples taken during this study were also analysed using a non-specific total protein tests to ensure that actual allergen removal was being measured and not merely a loss of ELISA immunoreactivity resulting from the aggressive cleaning interventions.

10.3 Results

Objective 1. All of the commercial ELISA kits used in this study produced 'broadly' similar results once the data had been normalised (see Fig. 1).
Objective 2. Peanut butter was generally more difficult to remove from all surfaces tested compared to hazelnut spread and milk custard.
Objective 3. Automated washing using a commercial dishwasher was generally more effective than manual washing with commercial detergents. Sponges were found to be the least effective cleaning material, and in terms of the comparison between detergents and hot water alone, there were differences, but those differences weren't significant for all surfaces.
Objective 4. There was no discernible difference between the ease of cleaning of different types of physical contact surfaces (stainless steel, High density polyethylene (HDPE), wood etc.).

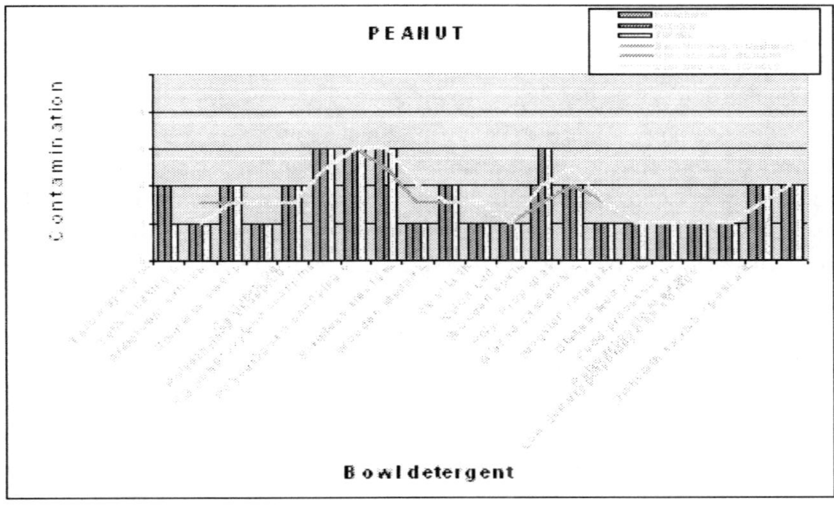

Fig. 10.1. Results for residual peanut protein using manual bowl washing

Having ascertained a number of key parameters (both physical and chemical) which influenced ease of cleaning, it was decided that further work be conducted to test the statistical relevance of these findings.

Peanut was selected as the allergenic simulant for further study as this had proved the most difficult to clean from all surfaces and the cleaning methods chosen were automated washing vs. manual bowl washing using a commercial detergent. The effectiveness of different commercial surface cleaners was also assessed. For both of these parameters the number of replicates was increased and the data was tested using statistical analysis software (SAS analysis).

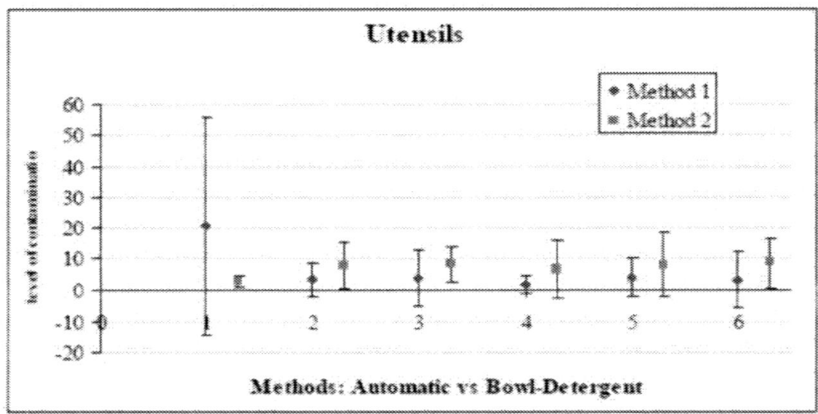

Fig. 10.2. Methods

Method 1 - Automated washing
Method 2 - Manual bowl washing

Results from the SAS analysis for different utensils, comparing the automated wash versus a bowl wash with commercial detergent showed differences for the majority of utensils. Automated washing in almost all cases was more effective in removing peanut from chopping boards and utensils when compared to bowl washing with detergents. There were however no significant differences in the effectiveness of different commercial surface cleaning products used, or between the different types of contact surfaces to which the peanut butter was applied (i.e. steel, nylon, polycarbonate, high density polyethylene, and wood). The findings of this study did broadly mirror the results and conclusions of study conducted in 2004 US schools (1).

To obtain a full copy of this report please contact the author.

10.4 References

1. Tamara T., Perry M.D. at col. Distribution of peanut allergen in the environment. *Journal of Allergy and Clinical Immunology.* 113 (5), 973-976 2004

11. PATTERNS AND PREVALENCE OF FOOD ALLERGY ACROSS EUROPE

Dr Clare Mills, Programme Leader
Food Structure and Health, Institute of Food Research

11.1 Introduction

The Institute of Food Research in Norwich leads the EuroPrevall study, which aims to collect information on the patterns and prevalence of food allergy across Europe and beyond. 30 years ago, no-one had ever heard of food allergies, and there certainly were not the headlines that appear in the newspapers about people dying from allergic reactions, and all the information that has appeared on food packaging about allergens. There certainly was not a need for children to be given adrenalin pens, nor were peanuts banned from entire schools because of children with peanut allergies. The question is, what has changed? Nowadays, many more people are interested in and informed about food allergy, but there are many more people who do not understand how awful an allergic reaction can be: how scary they are, that a bite of food can kill, a kiss from someone who has recently eaten an allergenic food can cause a reaction in someone allergic to that food. These are just examples of the sorts of reactions that can occur.

To protect these allergic people, the EuroPrevall project was started with the aim of studying how many people are affected, how geography affects risk and what levels of allergens provoke responses in those susceptible.

11.2 Definition of Food Allergy and Food Intolerance

There is a lot of confusion about what an allergy is, and what an intolerance is; these terms are often used indiscriminately. The European Academy of Allergy and Clinical Immunology classification of adverse reactions of foods was developed some years ago, and describes allergic reactions as non-toxic reactions to foods that are sub-divided into non immune-mediated food intolerance, and IgE- or non IgE-mediated food allergy. Non immune-mediated food intolerance can be enzymic, a good example of which is lactose intolerance, caused by a deficiency of lactase, and a lot of people who have milk intolerance actually have lactose intolerance. There can be pharmacological intolerances, such as those to amines that may trigger migraines. People can react to high levels of histamine in certain kinds of foods, and there are a host of other ill-defined reactions. There is one type of non-IgE mediated food allergy that is very well characterised, and is known as celiac disease or gluten intolerance.

The subject of this chapter is immune-mediated food allergy and its prevalence across Europe. An IgE-mediated reaction occurs when an allergen binds to IgE. IgE is a molecule that the body produces as part of its response to parasitic infections such as malaria, and sits on the surface of mast cells, which are packed full of histamine and other inflammatory mediators. When IgE comes into contact with the allergen, the allergen causes IgE molecules to cluster together on the surface of the mast cell, which causes the mast cell to de-granulate and release inflammatory mediators. It is those mediators that go on to cause the symptoms that we recognise as an allergic reaction.

11.3 Allergen Labelling in Europe

Europe is characterised by a history of consumer protection, and that behind the developments in allergen labelling can be traced back to proposals made by the Nordic countries in 1991 that ultimately led to FAO/WHO suggestions for inclusion of allergens on food labels. Most of the list of allergens that we currently use for allergen labelling was produced by a group of experts nearly 20 years ago, and one of the problems the food industry may have in the future is that the allergen labelling legislation has been framed on the basis of information that was available at that time, but does not consider more recent data about patterns and prevalence.

That allergen labelling list throws up lots of questions, for example: how will the list be modified objectively, whether allergens will be added to list, or allergens removed; how are allergens measured in food; analytical methods are important, and assay performance, is an issue; what allergens, and how much of the food supply should be tested; and how can the effects of processing be predicted effectively. One other thing that seems to have been overlooked, is an assessment of how much all the control of allergens and prevention of cross-contamination and appropriate allergen labelling is going to actually improve people's quality of life, because allergen management has a cost to the food industry.

11.4 The Cost of Food Allergy

To understand and manage food allergy, it is important to understand its scope, how much it costs the food industry to deal with it and also the cost to the allergic consumer. Certainly the intangible costs in terms of impact on quality of life are significant. This information is needed for policy makers, for health services for provision for chronic lifelong debilitating conditions, and ultimately research into developing preventive and curative strategies. The current situation is that if somebody has a food allergy all that doctors can say is “don’t eat a particular food” and give you an epipen in case you accidentally do. That really is not a very satisfactory state of affairs for anybody.

11.5 EuroPrevall

One of the objectives of the EuroPrevall project is to establish how many people suffer from food allergy in Europe, what the major foods causing food allergy are, what are the relationships between severity and minimum eliciting doses, how much of a food causes a problem, what is the impact on quality of life, how much does it cost to society, and what are the risk factors.

At the beginning of the project, state of the art papers were produced, including two papers that looked at the prevalence of food allergy and the data currently available. This is quite interesting and enlightening because prevalence figures are commonly used, such as between 1 to 7% of people have food allergy - where does that data come from? A systematic review was undertaken of studies of people with self-reported symptoms. This means that researchers have asked people whether they have a food allergy, without conducting clinical assessments to establish true, rather than perceived allergy. Depending on the study, the overall allergy prevalence varied between 3 and 35%. There are a smaller number of studies in which researchers asked whether people suffered from food allergy, and followed this up by checking whether those people who said they suffered from food allergy did in fact have symptoms, or had an IgE response, and there was a similar variation in prevalence between 3 and 35%.

The gold standard of diagnosing a food allergy is to actually feed someone the food that they are potentially allergic to. This type of investigation revealed a lower incidence of allergy, with overall allergy prevalence varying between 1 and 4%, for milk, eggs, fish and shellfish, but the data are very incomplete.

The general conclusions of this exercise were that food allergy determined in other studies is highly heterogeneous. This is partly due to variations in response rates, variations in diagnostic procedures and overall study design, and makes comparisons very difficult.

EuroPrevall aims to try and plug this data gap. This will be done over four and a half years, with 63 partners from 23 different countries, and collaborators all round the world including Africa, Asia, USA, Canada, New Zealand and Australia. The project will be investigating environmental, dietary and genetic influences on food allergy, and delivering information (patterns and prevalence, socioeconomic cost) and new tools to improve management. Foods studied by the project will be drawn from those included in the allergen labelling directive; eggs, milk, fish, shrimp, peanut, soya, hazelnut, walnut, wheat, celery, sesame and mustard. Other foods with differences in geographic distribution of allergy, for example peach, will also be studied. Peach allergy is a problem in the Mediterranean area, and it causes very severe reactions. Emerging foods causing allergic reactions, such as kiwi fruit will be included; kiwi was not part of the diet in the UK until 1972. There other new foods; buckwheat, and poppy seed, and the project will be looking at connections between pollen allergies, and allergies to fruit, and latex and allergies for example, to banana.

11.5.1 EuroPrevall population studies

EuroPrevall is using 3 complementary population studies. The first type, because there are different rates of food allergies in young children, is a birth cohort run in a number of different centres around Europe, including one in the UK funded by the Food Standards Agency. The idea behind this work is to capture the impact of maternal influences such as weaning on allergy incidence, and to record incidences of food allergy in children under 3 years old. This work is complemented by community surveys in unselected populations, run in some of the same centres that are running the birth cohort work These community surveys include school-age children (aged 8 – 12), and adults. This work will result in prevalence information. However it is very difficult to draw conclusions when research captures information on thousands and thousands of people; it tells you how many food allergic individuals there are, but may not provide hard data on the spread of incidence of allergies to different foods. The work is therefore complemented with an out-patient clinic study, which involves a self-selected population, because the people going into the out-patient clinic are the people who have gone to their doctor with a food allergy, and the patterns may be influenced to some extent by the health care system in a country. But nevertheless, that provides a large cohort of people with different types of food allergy. There are more than 4,000 babies in the birth cohort, and they will be followed to two and a half years within the current project, but it would be ideal to have more funding, because ultimately the power of the cohort is to carry on following these children up until they are 18 or 19 years old.

11.5.1.1 Birth cohort results

What has been found in the birth cohort, at about the age of 1 year is that the 2 dominant allergens are milk and egg and there is a small incidence of allergy to soya, some wheat, some peanuts and fish. In the UK cohort, there is one child who is allergic to broccoli which is very unusual. There are geographic differences. For example, in Germany, allergy relates mostly to cows milk with some peanut. In the UK, cows' milk and peanut are equally prevalent causes of allergy. In Greece, peanut allergy does not register at all, and that is a problem for the food industry in that allergy varies from country to country. The babies in the birth cohort are diagnosed with double blind placebo controlled food challenge (DBPCFC); the potentially allergenic food is disguised in another food. For babies it is actually in an infant formula, a highly hydrolysed product, or in a pudding. About half of the children were double blind positive. So a lot of information about cows' milk and egg allergy has been produced.

11.5.1.2 Community study results

In the community surveys for the school age children, researchers went into schools to assess children's allergy status. For adults, obtaining the sampling frame was more difficult. In Greece, for example, telephone surveys were used to recruit participants, and the target was around 3,000 subjects. Adults were asked to complete a short questionnaire, which contained a lot of questions based on many other studies that Peter Burney, who leads this project at Imperial College, has worked on to identify allergic individuals. These adult cases of food allergy are self-reported, and are people who think they have got a food allergy.

Respondents with self-reported allergy are asked to come to the clinic and given an extended questionnaire. A blood sample is taken, and that blood is used to determine whether there is IgE present in the sample that responds to lots of different foods. Those people who are what is called history positive, and IgE positive, then come in to the clinic, and they are fully evaluated and undergo a DBPCFC. As the study progresses the response rates get lower and lower because each series of tests takes more and more time. Nevertheless data is coming through from these community surveys.

What has been fascinating, and is the same as for the birth cohort, is the variation across Europe. Lithuania, Bulgaria, and Athens showed virtually no food allergy in adults. Utrecht in the Netherlands, and Zurich, had much higher levels of food allergy, so there are geographic differences in the patterns of allergies, and the incidence.

11.5.1.3 Out-patient clinic results

The out-patient clinic study in Madrid includes 2,000 patients who are recruited after they have come to the clinic looking for help with food allergy. These patients are asked to take part in the study, and undergo full clinical evaluation, and then have a double blind challenge to milk, egg, peanut, hazelnut, celery, apple, peach, fish and shrimp.

11.5.2 Allergenic foods

In terms of the number of people with confirmed IgE-mediated allergy, the most commonly noted foods are apple and hazelnut, followed by peanut, then peach, celery, fish and shrimp. In Europe these are referred to as *priority one* foods.

Something that we might not realise in the UK is that hazelnut is really important across Europe. Milk and egg allergy incidence is almost entirely in children.

Priority two foods include kiwi fruit and walnut. Kiwi is a significant allergen all across Europe. Quite a few people reported being allergic to soya, but there were very few people with confirmed allergy to it.

Priority three foods include carrot, which is a real problem in Lithuania, followed by tomato, melon, and banana. The tomato allergens are poorly characterised, but this is a significant allergenic food.

So there are foods here that are emerging as allergens, and certainly the top self-reported foods are hazelnut, apple, walnut, peanut, peach, and kiwi fruit, with similar trends in the out-patient and the community surveys.

This does cast doubt on the validity of the regulated list of major allergens that includes soya; there are not many people with soya bean allergy in this project, which includes thousands of people with food allergies. There are other very important allergenic foods, and for the fruit allergies it is a question of how the food industry would want to manage them, and indeed, whether they are a relevant concern for the food industry.

11.5.3 DBPCFC and threshold testing

The DBPCFC provides data on amounts of allergen prevalence, and data on how many people suffer from food allergy. Results show that prevalence differs around Europe, so in Utrecht it might be 2 or 3% of adults, but in Athens the incidence is low. So how do you set a prevalence rate for Europe? This is a challenge for Europe; how do we set one rate that covers everybody in a realistic way. The foods consumed between different countries are different. The next question is, how much food causes an allergic reaction?

EuroPrevall is using 2 common matrices to try and establish an eliciting dose for an allergen; one is a chocolate dessert matrix, and the other is a chocolate bar. It was not possible to eliminate the taste of shrimp in the chocolate dessert matrix, so shrimp burgers were used for that. The flavour of fish was eliminated in the chocolate dessert, however. The protocol has been designed to give what is called a no effect level. When somebody comes in to the clinic, they do not know what they will be given: one day they will eat the active dose, one day the placebo; they do not know which dose they are going to eat, and the person giving them the challenge does not know what they are eating either. Participants are observed while they eat increasing amounts, starting from 3 micrograms of allergenic protein, and researchers are able to calculate that back into what it means in terms of a peanut or a fish etc. Patients carry on consuming low-dose challenges eating gradually larger and larger amounts of the allergenic protein, and the idea is that the top dose is a daily serving (3 g of protein), but with shrimp, researchers were having to give so much shrimp protein that actually the top level doses are open challenges with up to half a dozen prawns. As someone is given the doses, there is a twenty-minute interval between the doses, and the clinicians watch the patient, and note the symptoms, and the symptoms are scored either as subjective or objective. Subjective symptoms are those where, for example, the patient feels a tingling feeling, or feels sick or dizzy. Objective symptoms include skin rashes, changes in asthma, urticaria, rhinitis, conjunctivitis etc.

For cows' milk challenges, skimmed milk powder is used as the active ingredient. There is currently double blind challenge threshold data for around 60 people, a lot of whom are children, less than 5 years, and they have been done with the bottled milk in the sinlak product. Quite a few school age children are allergic to cows' milk, and only a small number of adults with cows milk allergy, which have been tested with the chocolate dessert.

For testing with hens' egg, pasteurised egg white was used. The reason is that very few egg yolk allergens have ever been described, and blinding egg yolk causes problems because it produces odd flavours. The main foods causing allergies in young infants were cows' milk and egg, and gave objective symptoms at low doses in the oral challenges. These data confirm the importance of these allergens, especially since they present the food industry with particular management problems because of the powdered nature in which they are used.

To test for fish, freeze-dried cod powder that was specially prepared by AgriFood Canada was used, and there may be thirty patients in total who will have a positive challenge. Quite a few of these, about 9, will come from the birth cohort, and the rest will probably be school age children and adults.

So far there are 15 patients who have reacted to shrimp, and it may be that the project will have to supplement this with challenges that will be done in Hong Kong, because there is a huge amount of shellfish, crab, and lobster allergy in Asia.

Interestingly enough in Europe, people who react to fish and shrimp are predominantly from Iceland and Greece. Low dose subjective challenges of 3 micrograms of protein were used, but many of the patients needed to eat very large amounts of allergen to actually give an objective reaction. This is the case where open challenges of whole prawns have had to be used.

There are many patients that react to plant foods, including hazelnut; there are more people allergic to hazelnut than any other food in the study. There will be a lot of threshold data on hazelnut, including people who have nut allergies that we might expect to see in the UK, but also the kind of hazelnut allergies that are associated with birch pollen allergy.

Peanuts are producing fascinating results; peanuts are given in exactly the same base matrix as the other allergens. It has actually been very difficult to get even 28 positive challenges, and the target is 30 positive challenges, but it has proven very difficult, and this is because whilst we might see peanut allergy here in the UK and it might occur in Canada or even in Australia, in mainland Europe peanut allergy is not a big issue.

Celeriac or, celery spice has over 40 patients who have had a positive reaction, including school age children and adults consuming the dessert matrix, and one of the things found in Europe relating to this, is that this is not simply a Swiss problem, but it is a central European problem and occurs in Poland and Lithuania.

Soya has had hardly any patients with a positive reaction, and these are almost all from the birth cohort.

The EuroPrevall project will run to the end of 2009, and the next question is, what are we going to do with all the data? A workshop 2 years ago with the Food Standards Agency in Madrid produced a paper that is looking at the framework for managing the way forward, and one of the important uses of this information is probabilistic risk assessment; this is an example of how information from different strands of research are needed in order to take a probabilistic view of who is going to have an allergic reaction. Work is ongoing with the FSA looking at tolerable risks; how many people can be effectively protected within this population. EuroPrevall will provide a lot of the data on thresholds that will be needed for these risk calculations, as will the Food Allergy Research and Resource Programme (FARRP) run from the University of Nebraska. In another two years there will have been progress made on thresholds.

So going forward, we do need to look for future work to develop realistic robust management strategies that protect the allergic consumers without restricting food choice or imposing ridiculous burdens on our food manufacturers, and to actually develop improved analytical methods and performance.

Acknowledgements

This work was funded by the EU through the EuroPrevall project (FOOD-CT-2005-514000) and the BBSRC through an Institute Strategic Programme Grant to IFR. Thanks go to Phil Johnson for editorial comments.

12. ALLERGENS - THE MOST VULNERABLE AREAS OF A FOOD FACTORY

Jeremy Hall, Group Technical Director,
Bernard Matthews Farms

12.1 Introduction

This chapter will give manufacturers a view on how the most vulnerable areas of food factories should be managed – in this case, food allergens. There are probably at least 20 major vulnerabilities within a manufacturing facility. These include people, engineers, product development and most of the manufacturing managers and supervisors are all a risk.

12.2 Allergen Management

A company should understand what allergens are held on its sites. Without that knowledge, allergen management is very difficult. There should be a risk analysis conducted on each of those allergens, and there should be an assessment within the operational areas that are used, regarding how they are used, whether they need to be used in that way, and all the pre-held conditions and pre-held conceptions should be challenged.

Management and staff knowledge are vital to allergen management.

Effective planning falls within the role of the planning department, who decide how manufacturing will be done, and their ability to understand and work within, and accept and understand the requirements that technical staff are placing upon them in terms of manufacturing goods in a safe, planned and effective manner.

Raw material sourcing is also a very important area of consideration, and will be discussed in detail in this chapter.

Other possible transfers of allergy risk arise from moving allergens from an area where they are controlled, into an area where they should not be present, or where they may not be controlled at all.

The possible allergens held on site may include peanuts, which at the moment are considered to be one of the high profile allergens, as much because of the impact that nuts tend to have on those that are allergic to them. Tree nuts, milk and dairy products, eggs, fish, crustaceans soya, wheat, celery, sesame, sulphur dioxide, and lupin, are all on the mandatory list of allergens that should be labelled, and of course one material that is a non food allergen, but one that companies should be aware of in food factories, is latex in terms of latex in gloves worn by people handling food during manufacture.

When assessing and reducing the risks from allergens in a business, simplification of the process is the key. A Company should check how many of the allergens are used within a facility, and what shared risks do they have. Within that assessment, what the team at Bernard Matthews has tended to do is to challenge the whole preconception in terms of the risks from allergens that there are in the business. How the manufacturing and planning of products is colour coded is assessed, together with looking closely at which of the allergenic ingredients there are on site, where they are in which parts of the facility, and trying to make sure that everyone within that facility understands the risks and that controlling allergen contamination is the primary factor. At Bernard Matthews it was found that manufacturing goods in a scaled manner worked well, so that products that are made at the beginning of a shift in each area have zero allergen content, and production progresses through the day with consideration of the addition of allergens into manufacturing facilities in a controlled manner, assuming that the business accepts use of those allergens at all.

12.3 Allergen Removal

A fairly crucial question is whether allergens need to be used in products at all. It is important first to challenge all areas of a business, whether the allergens currently being used are actually needed, or can they be substituted with other non-allergenic ingredients. Can specifications and systems be reviewed, with a view to reducing the amount of allergens in your products and on your site? Obviously this isn't always possible; if you are producing chocolate, you are obliged to use milk. Bernard Matthews produces a lot of breaded poultry products, so there is wheat and other allergens in those areas. Controlling a known allergen is one thing, running the risk of transfers from other parts of the factory, and from other risk areas is another thing. NPD teams may be able to reformulate some of your products to remove those allergens completely. It's the simplest way of reducing risk, although most NPD teams don't like being challenged in this way, and take it somewhat personally when they are asked to remove allergens from a product. However an NPD team is part of the same team effort, and it is important to get them onside and working to help reduce allergen risk; substituting allergenic for non-allergenic ingredients in a formulation is one of the quickest and easiest ways of having a real impact. Once that stage has been accomplished, the remaining task is to consider how to manage those risks that are left.

At Bernard Matthews nearly all the allergens have been removed from areas where it was felt that they weren't necessary, and this was achieved without any major change to the products; it was just a matter of finding alternative ingredients that delivered the same benefits.

12.4 Staff Training and Supplier Audits

Management and staff knowledge is one of the biggest areas that companies need to work on, individually, and as an industry. On visiting supplying factories to find out what the level of allergen knowledge is, the technical teams at supplying companies tend to understand allergen management, and some of the managers, but not all have got a good grasp of it, and that's really where the weakness can come in. Responsibility therefore, both within your own manufacturing facility, and in all the supplying companies that you draw ingredients from, must be held, understood and adopted fully. Managers within your own business should be assessed, to ensure that they are being trained adequately to work within the risk presented by the product ranges that they are handling within that site. They need to understand the implications of accidental contamination, and to understand that allergens can actually injure and kill people, sometimes with long term injuries even if affected consumers don't die.

A company should look at how much training is in place, and at what level of detail? Who does the training? Drawing upon the expertise of staff from Campden BRI and Leatherhead Food Research to train your staff is a very useful plan, especially to draw in senior management to the site, to educate them on allergen management and risk, and in the process to cascade that knowledge down through further training using your onsite training teams.

The knowledge being passed on to those that are handling these products is the essential component, and without effectively passing the knowledge onto the factory floor, then risks will certainly be present. So you have got to ask, do your line supervisors understand fully the risks they are dealing with? It is very difficult to argue that due diligence is anywhere near adequate unless the people that are handling the foods at all places down the line fully understand what they are doing and how things need to be done. Are your controls firmly in place? A company should be looking at every person involved in the manufacturing process within a facility. Whether a company is buying ingredients or manufacturing, they should know that the controls are firmly in place and won't be bypassed, and the whole attitude within the business should be one of protection of the end consumer, and therefore making sure that the accidental use of an allergen, or the failure to completely clean an facility cannot be allowed to happen.

Is allergen control driven into and through the company? It is very important that a company fully gets to grips with the knowledge of allergen controls. This applies to people who are onsite, and those that are not onsite, and staff should understand what is required, and if challenged by visitors, such as auditors from outside the business, they should be able to demonstrate clear, concise and adequate knowledge on what the risks are.

In the past Bernard Matthews has engaged in discussion with potential suppliers of ingredients, and are presented with lists of audits and approvals that these companies have, but when a factory visit takes place, don't always find that those audits and approvals really give the level of protection that we think is necessary to make sure that the risks are at the lowest possible standard, and really are very pleased and impressed to see under version 5 of the BRS Standard that allergens is involved a lot more. Bernard Matthews think that this is an essential area and wholeheartedly agree with the comment that the one-up and one-down approach in terms of traceability and knowledge of where ingredients have come from is not a due diligence defence. Bernard Matthews would certainly expect to challenge any supplier of ingredients to us that they know where the ingredients have come from, and the sources of the materials they have used to manufacture those products. A Company must be sure that they know what they are bringing into their manufacturing facility, because otherwise they may accidentally bring in something that they do not wish to be present on their site. Companies need to know how their suppliers operate in detail, and this can only be done by getting inside your suppliers, and in the same way that retailers come to audit the Bernard Matthews manufacturing facilities, Bernard Matthews visit its suppliers, and are very thorough in their inspections.

If a Company is handling allergenic ingredients on its facility at all, it may potentially be delisted as a supply source if it is a high risk ingredient. Bernard Matthews is very sensitive about nut ingredients on sites of its suppliers, and try to make sure that risks are minimised, by putting in the right sort of safety procedures in terms of its supply base.

Do other companies carry out detailed supplier audits, and third party supplier audits? These are recommended in order to properly understand how allergens are handled. If BRC systems and other audit systems develop to the point where one has faith in them, then they should be adopted. It's a costly exercise, but then what is the cost to company image, brand, and product if a mistake happens.

12.5 Assessing Risk from Production Machinery

In terms of facilities on your site, if you look at the complexity of the machines; most manufacturing facilities are using conveyors. It is virtually impossible to clean a conveyor and remove egg protein. Bernard Matthews have tried to do this, repeated tests have been done, and methodologies have been discussed, including using chemicals, hot water etc. Very few of these systems in a manufacturing operation can effectively remove the protein to the point where there will be a negative result from a test. In terms of the machines used on some sites, for example a tumbling unit, there are so many nooks and crannies in that type of equipment, that it isn't possible to do an effective clean, particularly in the middle of a manufacturing shift, so that any allergens that were used earlier in the day cannot be removed without a thorough clean down. This is where effective planning has to come into force; managers need to make sure that the people that are planning to change facilities in a manufacturing plant understand the risks and what they are doing in altering the order of production runs, because with special promotions such as Buy One Get One Free's, and other promotions, there is a tremendous commercial pressure coming through from your customer base to complete an order in full, and perhaps encouraging someone to bypass some of the controls is a real risk in your factory.

So, scaling production in relation to the allergenic risks is the logical way forward, and it is one of the few ways that risk can be effectively minimised.

The practicalities of the cleaning procedures are assessed in each of the areas, and between production processes. A company should be asking, can it deliver the level of safety that is needed. In many cases, this is a tall order, and companies should be looking at designating specific areas for handling specific products. Egg residue is a classic example of accepting that there is a risk in a particular area, and managing the products that are made in that area accordingly. Hot water, detergent, sanitizers and even repeated CIP systems won't remove all of the allergens on a slow basis, or a standard clean.

So a Company should decide how to operate with the allergens present, work out ways to do it in the safest manner possible and also of course make sure that you are labelling your products adequately, effectively and continuously, and announcing the allergen status of your products to any consumers that are going to buy your products.

12.6 Raw Material Sourcing

Raw material sourcing is one of the most important areas of allergen management. For raw material sourcing, Bernard Matthews has started to install a new product development computerised system through Siemens. The aim of it is specifically to share data around a much wider group of people within the company, and those involved will include product development, raw material purchasing teams, manufacturing teams that will be involved in the early stages of production trials, and full technical and QA teams. By sharing that information, and by making sure that everybody is aware of new ingredients that are going to be potentially purchased, potentially sourced and put into trial operations, challenges can be built into this type of system that try and prevent some of the occurrences that would otherwise potentially happen where people buy in raw materials from small sources, don't do adequate evaluations, and don't draw up a detailed enough specification before it ends up as a product development issue.

12.7 Other Possible Transfers of Allergenic Risk

In theory, every one of your machine parts and where your food ingredients come into contact are risk areas. Each one should be inspected, and a risk assessment should be done, and they should be built into HACCP plans. This is second nature to most companies, but manufacturers should make sure that all ingredients suppliers are acting in the same way; and some do, others do not.

Areas of allergen transfer cannot be neglected; they must be factored into an allergen management plan to ensure that all the risks have been considered, and at all times should be built into risk analysis. In terms of lack of hygiene procedures in plant, the potential consequences of a lapse in hygiene should also be considered; the ease of spreading sesame seeds is well accepted. On a visit to a bakery section and having being told that, no, no, we don't have any of the allergens on site other than those that one would normally expect to find in a bread making facility, inspectors entered an adjacent area half an hour later that was considered to be a separate facility, but was located directly next the other facility, there was lots of sesame seed on various trays and on floors. On looking further it could be observed that sesame seeds had been walked from one side of the dividing wall to the other plant, completely outwitting the function of having separate facilities.

With respect to allergen transfer on clothes, don't ever think it can't happen, because that's the most likely time that that is exactly what will happen. Many manufacturers ban chocolate bars containing nuts in their canteens, and companies also need to educate staff not to bring such products onto site. Nuts are used in breakfast cereals, and in confectionery, and in terms of the minimising the risk of accidental contamination companies really have to make sure that their site is as free from risk as possible, and removing the possibility of these allergens accidentally being dropped into products is a must.

Cross-contamination from nearby production lines can also be a problem. If the system in question involves product that is being pumped through a high-pressure system there have to be measures in place to ensure that aerosols cannot escape and be blown from one side of the manufacturing facility to another. The dusting materials for crisps are easily transferred, and in some cases this may not present an undue risk, if the materials concerned do not contain allergens, but there are circumstances whereby materials can be moved from one manufacturing site to another, or one manufacturing line to another within a single air space.

Any machinery that can potentially leak material, whether it be milk, egg or any other ingredient, should be closely monitored, because that material can easily be moved around a factory unless it is controlled. Bernard Matthews certainly works on the basis that manufacturing lines that are using allergens are not to be used for alternative products just to try and take that one risk out of the process.

INDEX